SOCIAL AND PO

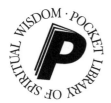

Practical Applications

Also in this series:

RUDOLF STEINER

SOCIAL AND POLITICAL SCIENCE

An Introductory Reader

Compiled with an introduction, commentary and notes by Stephen E. Usher

Sophia Books

All translations revised by Christian von Arnim

Sophia Books
An imprint of Rudolf Steiner Press
Hillside House, The Square
Forest Row, RH18 5ES

www.rudolfsteinerpress.com

Published by Rudolf Steiner Press 2003

For earlier English publications of individual selections please
see p. 209

The material by Rudolf Steiner was originally published in
German in various volumes of the 'GA' (*Rudolf Steiner
Gesamtausgabe* or Collected Works) by Rudolf Steiner Verlag,
Dornach. This authorized volume is published by permission of
the Rudolf Steiner Nachlassverwaltung, Dornach (for further
information see p. 214)

This edition translated © Rudolf Steiner Press 2003

All rights reserved. No part of this publication may be
reproduced, stored in a retrieval system, or transmitted, in any
form or by any means, electronic, mechanical, photocopying
or otherwise, without the prior permission of the publishers

A catalogue record for this book is available from the British
Library

ISBN 1 85584 103 7

Cover by Andrew Morgan Design
Typeset by DP Photosetting, Aylesbury, Bucks.
Printed and bound in Great Britain by Cromwell Press Limited,
Trowbridge, Wilts.

Contents

Introduction: Seminal Ideas and Historic Moments

by Stephen Usher

Rudolf Steiner (1861–1925) is best remembered today for establishing Waldorf education, a movement which has produced hundreds of schools around the world for children from kindergarten to school-leaving age. His reputation was different immediately after the First World War when he was recognized throughout Europe and the United States as a social thinker who had proposed an alternative to both communism and capitalism as a path for the reconstruction of post-war Central Europe. One British commentator, writing in the *London Quarterly Review*, stated that Steiner's book *Towards Social Renewal* was 'perhaps the most widely read of all books on politics appearing since the war'.[1] That book was also reviewed in significant places in the US such as the *New York Times Review of Books*, *Journal of Political Economy*, and *The American Economic Review*.[2]

Of course the twentieth century witnessed the struggle of capitalism versus communism to become the model for human social organization. When the Berlin Wall fell in 1989, capitalism was declared the victor, a notion trumpeted particularly by Francis Fukuyama in his *End of History and the Last Man*. The struggle between those two world views left little room for awareness of a third alternative during the course of the last century, particularly as Steiner's ideas lacked a 'laboratory' to unfold themselves.

But the victory of capitalism is hollow for it has failed to deliver even a tolerable material existence to much of the earth's population, to say nothing of a more spiritual sense of fulfilment. For this reason it seems appropriate to bring before the public today this selection of Steiner's social ideas, which are like seeds from some Vavilovian centre that have lain dormant for many years but still retain their power of germination. They offer something vital to humanity's social thinking, which has grown sterile over the long course of the twentieth century.

The selection is arranged chronologically. It begins with the 24-year-old Steiner's discussion of the difference between the methods of the life sciences and the social sciences from 'Psychological cognition', a chapter of his *A Theory of Knowledge Based on Goethe's World Conception*. His 1898 article from *Das Magazin für Literatur*, entitled 'The social question', is the second selection. Here Steiner develops what he calls the fundamental sociological law: 'In the early stages of cultural evolution, mankind tends towards the formation of social units; initially the interests of individuals are sacrificed to the interests of those groupings; the further progress of development leads to the emancipation of the individual from the interests of the groupings and to the unrestricted development of needs and capacities of the individual.' He describes the goal and social ideal of this evolution as 'anarchistic individualism'.

In 1905 Steiner wrote an essay titled 'The science of the spiritual and the social question'[3] in which he develops what is for him a fundamental social law: 'The well-being of a total community of human beings working together becomes greater the less the individual demands the products of his achievements for himself, that is, the more of these products he passes on to his fellow workers and the more his own needs are not satisfied out of his own achievements, but out of the achievements of others.' On 26 October 1905, he delivered a lecture titled 'The social question and theosophy' where he develops the same set of concepts using different examples, and it is this lecture that is our third selection.

It is worth observing that on 26 July 1922, when he delivered the cycle of lectures published under the title *World Economy*,[4] Steiner commented about this fundamental social law that 'it would only have had real significance if it had been taken up by men of affairs and if they had acted accordingly. But it was left altogether unnoticed; consequently I did not complete it or publish any more of it.' He proceeded, in these lectures of 1922, to link the concept of the division of labour to his concept of the fundamental social law, showing that when economic production was dominated by large-scale division of labour the law was achieved, in a certain sense, because then the worker in what he is actually doing is literally providing for the needs of others far more than is the case in more primitive economic conditions. (A worker on an assembly line, perhaps, stamps a single piece of metal thousands of times per day and these go into thousands of cars that meet the needs of thousands of people all around the world. By contrast, in a primitive community a person spends part of his time farming and part of his time spinning yarn, which meets his own needs and that of his immediate family and perhaps, through barter, the needs of a few more people in his immediate circle.) From this fact flows the great vitality of the modern economic process, but this vitality is contradicted by the selfish motivation that brings people to work. A particularly clear explanation of how Steiner's threefold social organization would make possible a different type of motivation to work is found in the collection of Steiner's newspaper articles of the early 1920s published under the title *Renewal of the Social Organism*.[5] The argument is ably summarized in Joseph Weizenbaum's foreword to this volume.

Steiner's 'law of true price', which he first formulated in a footnote to *Towards Social Renewal*[6] (1919) and elaborated in the lecture of 29 July 1922 in *World Economy*, is also closely related to his fundamental social law. Indeed, the law of true price is a way of bringing about the fundamental social law in an economy based on market prices in such a way that both the actual production and the motivation to work are consistent with the law and that maximum anarchical individualism is possible. Steiner states the law of true price as follows: 'A true price is forthcoming when a man receives, as counter-value for the product he has made, sufficient to enable him to satisfy the whole of his needs, including of course the needs of his dependants, until he will again have completed a like product.'[7]

From these brief comments one gets a glimpse of how Steiner first developed his observations about the fundamental social law in seed form and how after an interval of 14 years he returned to it again and showed how the idea expanded and developed like a plant that metamorphoses from seed to leaf to blossom. During the period between 1905 and the outbreak of the First World War in 1914, Steiner said little about social issues, at least in a direct way. Then in 1915 he returned to social concerns with his essay 'Thoughts during the time of war, to the Germans and those who do not believe they have to hate them.'[8]

It was in June and July of 1917 that he introduced his seminal idea of the threefold social order. He developed the idea in response to the question of Otto Lerchenfeld (1868–1938), who worked in the Berlin government during these difficult war years. Lerchenfeld came to Steiner with the question: Is there any way out of the catastrophic situation that has engulfed Europe? (The war had raged for three long years and, before it was over, more than 30 million people had died.) Steiner responded by giving Lerchenfeld a three-week private seminar on the threefold social order. Lerchenfeld gave a brief description of his experience in his memoirs, as follows:

> More than three weeks of day-long, hour-long work followed this first conference. They were weeks of the loftiest experience, the highest tension, the most intense learning; learning what logic of life is in truth; learning of becoming and fading away; learning how logic must encompass life in an artistic way; learning how it must not weaken upon contact with real life and become illogical. Politics is art and not science alone. When it is only mere science it makes the social organism ill because the organism is then handled as a dead thing.
>
> And then one beautiful day the complete structure was there, put together stone upon stone in the utmost detail. There was nothing of the abstract, no theory, no programme, nothing merely thought out. These have nothing to do with the onward movement of life. In the building of this structure, on the other hand, every one of the weighty relations of life was asked, as it were: 'What do you need, and you and you, in order to prosper as freely, joyfully, and soundly as possible and to become what you might become and ought to become if you are to be able to fulfil your mission in the totality

of the social order?' And the answers of all, as if bound together in a garland, did not provide what was intended to become a definitive solution of the social question, and could naturally not be this by reason of the very nature of a living organism. Nevertheless, there did result out of this idea the way, the only straightforward way upon which the social conditions, the social difficulties with their eternally varying problems, might be guided again and again towards a solution appropriate to the period, towards their curing.[9]

Following this seminar, Steiner developed a plan together with Lerchenfeld and Ludwig Polzer-Hoditz (1869–1945) to bring about an armistice on the condition that Central Europe be permitted to reconstruct itself on the basis of the threefold social order. As such it was an alternative to the idea of a 'peace without victory'[10] then being circulated by the American president Woodrow Wilson.

To bring about this plan Steiner drafted his two memoranda of 1917 and these two memoranda constitute the next item presented in this collection. They are not easy reading for contemporaries because they are directed to the senior statesmen of the Austro-Hungarian Empire and of the Germany of that day. As such they assume a reader intimately familiar with the history of those regions, including all the important events of the war and its outbreak. Naturally they also assume a reader familiar with the state structures of these countries at that time.

In addition to introducing the concept of the threefold social order, the memoranda offered the statesmen a perspective on the outbreak of the war and where lay responsibility for that catastrophe; on the manner in which the British were managing war propaganda to their extreme advantage; and on esoteric considerations about the geo-political aspirations of the Anglo-American world and how these worked into the war. The memoranda really should be read together with two other documents that were known to Steiner and that support the position he took in the memoranda.[11] The first is the 1914 memoir on the outbreak of the war[12] written by Helmuth von Moltke, chief-of-staff of the German army at the outbreak of the war. This provides a unique insight into the state of the German leadership at that time and supports Steiner's thesis that Germany was not solely responsible for the war, a view which is contrary to the weight of historical opinion and the clause of the Treaty of Versailles attributing sole guilt to the Germans.[13]

In particular, von Moltke's memoir presents a symptomatological picture of the whole illness of the German leadership.[14] Von Moltke describes how Kaiser Wilhelm briefly halted western mobilization of the German army due to a mistaken hope that the British were about to agree to remain neutral and guarantee that the French would not attack. Given the precision timing and coordination required in those times to mobilize an army of one million soldiers, interfering with the mobilization was extremely risky as it could have brought about complete chaos with catastrophic consequences for Germany. That the mobilization was halted indicates how little the political leadership understood the military's Schlieffen Plan that was the only military option available.[15] That plan called for a rapid dual front assault to the west and the east and was created out of an understanding of the complex treaties that governed international relations at the time. The treaty between the Russians and the French, in particular, required both to go to the defence of the other if war broke out. While the halt demonstrated that the political leadership was out of touch with reality when it entertained the idea that the British would give such a guarantee, it also shows that they were not hell bent on a two-front war and thus supports Steiner's contention that the British bore part of the responsibility for the western war as they could have prevented it by making the guarantee.

When confronted with the Kaiser's decision, von Moltke was greatly disturbed because he understood the implications of halting the mobilization and he entertained no delusions that such a guarantee would be forthcoming from England. In his memoir von Moltke explained how he argued that the mobilization should not be halted but rather carried forward so that the western part of the mobilization stop at the western German frontier. Then, if the guarantee were made, troops could be shifted to the east to counter the Russian mobilization that already was underway. Several hours after the Kaiser had called for the halt of the mobilization he received a telegram from his cousin, the King of England, advising that England would make no such guarantee. At this point the Kaiser summoned von Moltke and told him that he could do as he pleased.

This bizarre incident should be recognized for its value as a historical symptom. It is a historic experiment that reveals the intentions and confusion of the Kaiser and German government at the outbreak of the war. To use modern language, it is an asset-backed demonstration that they would not have invaded Belgium or France if they had received the British guarantee. Historians have largely ignored this remarkable piece of evidence.

Without the evidence of this symptom one might dismiss the conversation between the German ambassador to England, Lichnowsky, and the British Foreign Minister (Grey) as posturing on the part of the Germans, suggesting as Grey did that the ambassador was not speaking on behalf of his government. This conversation, which is itself another important symptom, is preserved in an official British telegram from Grey to the British ambassador to Berlin, Goschen:

I told the German ambassador today that the reply of the German government with regard to the neutrality of Belgium affected feeling in this country. If Germany could see her way to give the same assurances as that which had been given by France it would materially contribute to relieve anxiety and tension here. On the other hand, if there were a violation of the neutrality of Belgium by one combatant while the other respected it, it would be extremely difficult to restrain public feeling in this country. I said that we had been discussing this question at a Cabinet meeting, and, as I was authorized to tell him this, I gave him an *aide-mémoire* of it.

He asked me whether, if Germany gave a promise not to violate Belgian neutrality, we would engage to remain neutral.

I replied that I could not say that; our hands were still free, and we were considering what our attitude should be. All I could say was that our attitude would be determined largely by public opinion[16] here, and that the neutrality of Belgium would appeal very strongly to public opinion here. I did not think that we could give a promise of neutrality on that condition alone.

The Ambassador pressed me as to whether I could not formulate conditions on which we would remain neutral. He even suggested that the integrity of France and her colonies might be guaranteed.

I said that I felt obliged to refuse definitely any promise to remain neutral on similar terms, and I could only say that we must keep our hands free.[17]

The second item that deserves to be read together with Steiner's memoranda is the book *The Transcendental Universe: Six lectures on Occult Science, Theosophy and the Catholic Faith* by C.G. Harrison.[18] This volume was originally published in 1894 in England and it gives a unique look into the esoteric knowledge alive in England at the time and supports some of the statements made by Steiner in the memoranda.

Before leaving the theme of the Harrison book and Steiner's remarks in the memoranda about the secret societies that worked behind the scenes of the British and American governments, it should also be remarked that Steiner was highly critical of what developed in Germany after 1871.[19] In his preface to the von Moltke memoir Steiner argues that Germany had no business aspiring to become a world power based on 'exercise of power'. Rather it should have developed itself along a line consistent with its pre-1871 history as a cultural power as reflected, for example, in the idealist philosophers, Goethe, Schiller, the great musicians etc.[20] That was its rightful path of development. It also should be made clear that Steiner was not in sympathy with German nationalists. Indeed, Hitler attacked Steiner in print in 1921 and, in 1922, the early nationalists attempted to kill Steiner in Munich.[21]

The thrust of Steiner's advice in the memoranda to the Central European statesmen is that they should find the courage to proclaim to the world that they intended to move Central Europe forward, beyond the war, with the threefold social order as the organizational principle. According to Steiner the very appearance of this concept, issuing from the governing power of Central Europe, would paralyse the esoteric ambitions of the hidden Anglo-American establishment. Had they found the courage to follow this advice they would have brought about a legitimate and balancing centre between West and East that would have allowed a much healthier evolution of mankind over the twentieth century. Steiner's objective in giving this advice to the statesmen was to put Germany back on the course of its pre-1871 development. He viewed his threefold social order as arising from the real thread of middle European cultural development and history.

With the help of Ludwig Poltzer-Hoditz, Otto Lerchenfeld and others, the memoranda reached the hands of leading statesmen in Germany and Austro-Hungary. Ludwig Polzer-Hoditz had a brother, Arthur, who was the private secretary to the young emperor, Karl, of Austro-Hungary and through that channel Karl received a copy of the memoranda. But Karl never managed to pay sufficient attention to the ideas until it was too late.[22]

The memoranda also reached Prince Max von Baden who had several private conversations with Steiner on the topic of the threefold social order.[23] This happened prior to the end of the war when von Baden was made Imperial Chancellor by Kaiser Wilhelm and charged with nego-

tiating an armistice. Steiner had hoped that von Baden
would put forth the threefold idea as an alternative to
Woodrow Wilson's 14-point programme. But at the last
minute von Baden lost courage and on 5 October 1918 he
accepted the Wilson programme as the basis of an
armistice. Steiner refers to this failure in his 1919 book
Towards Social Renewal with these words, '[T]he terrible
spiritual capitulation came, brought on by a man in whom
many in German lands had placed something like a last
hope.'[24,25]

With von Baden's failure there was no further hope that
the threefold idea would be proposed to the world by
Central European governments as the basis for an armistice. Steiner consequently turned his attention to bringing
the idea to the grassroots in Central Europe. In his further
attempts to promote the idea of the threefold social order
Steiner never again referred to the secret esoteric circles of
the Anglo-American world in such a direct fashion as he
had done in the memoranda, as there was no longer any
reason to do so. The only possibility of creating a
countervailing power had been destroyed.[26] Moreover,
Steiner recognized that the leadership of the historic
evolution of mankind had passed into the hands of the
West and that civilization would only be prevented from
ruin if the English-speaking world could find the insight
to pour spirit into the economic impulses that it would
pursue.[27]

The last three items in our selection can be viewed as

part of this effort to stimulate a grassroots interest in the threefold idea, which also included his widely circulated 'Appeal to the German People'.[28] This was circulated as a newspaper insert by the hundreds of thousands across Central Europe in March of 1919. This effort also included the publication of Steiner's *Towards Social Renewal* in April of 1919.

In two of the remaining selections of this volume Steiner describes his own insights into the esoteric make-up of the peoples of the West, the East and the middle. Here he tries to convey his understanding of the idiosyncratic characteristics of different parts of the globe at the time which he felt needed to be understood by the peoples of the world if they were ever to live in harmony with one another. The remaining chapter of this volume, 'Culture, Law and Economics', is a newspaper article Steiner wrote at the end of 1919 when he was attempting to gain grassroots support for his threefold idea. It gives what is for my mind a particularly clear, short statement of the central idea.

1. Psychological Cognition

'Psychological Cognition' is a chapter from Rudolf Steiner's first book, A Theory of Knowledge Based on Goethe's World Conception.[29] *Steiner wrote this work when he was 24 years of age. An earlier section of the book is an enquiry regarding the difference between the sciences that study inorganic nature and those that study organic nature. Steiner argues that the study of organic nature already requires a kind of consciousness that transcends what is needed to study the dead world. Moreover, modern civilization is based on the type of consciousness that is appropriate for penetrating the laws of the dead world. To grasp the world of living things already requires stepping beyond the consciousness of our time. He develops the concept of the 'type' as the way to approach the living world. The following section of the book is titled, 'The spiritual or cultural sciences'. It is in this section that the chapter presented here is found. This section concerns itself with a form of consciousness that transcends what is needed to grasp the living world. It is what is needed to penetrate into the lawfulness of the world of ensouled beings. This realm includes what we know as psychology, sociology, political science, economics and history.*

The first science in which the human spirit deals with itself is psychology. The mind here stands observing itself.

Fichte assigned an existence to the human being only to the extent that the human being ascribes this to himself. In other words, human personality has only those traits, characteristics, capacities which it ascribes to itself through insight into its own being. A human capacity of which the human being knew nothing would not be recognized by him as his own but would be attributed to someone alien to him. When Fichte supposed that he could base the whole knowledge of the universe on this truth, he was in error. It is appropriate to be the highest principle of psychology. It determines the method of psychology. If the human spirit possesses a characteristic only in so far as it attributes this to itself, then the psychological method consists in the immersion of the mind in its own activity. Here, then, self-apprehension is the method.

It is obvious that in this discussion we do not restrict psychology to being the science of the accidental characteristics of any single (this one or that one) human individual. We release the single mind from its accidental limitations, from its accessory traits, and seek to raise ourselves to a consideration of the human individual as such.

Indeed, the key is not that we consider the wholly accidental single individuality but that we understand the self-determining individual as such. Whoever says at this point that in that case we are dealing with nothing more than the type of humanity confuses the type with the generalized concept. It is essential to the type that it, as the general, confronts its single forms. Not so with the concept of the human individual. Here the general is active directly in the individual being, except that this activity expresses itself in various ways according to the object towards which it is directed. The type exists in single forms and in these enters into reciprocal activity with the external world. The human spirit has only one form. But in one set of circumstances certain objects move his feelings; in another an ideal inspires him to action etc. It is not a specialized form of the human spirit; it is always the entire and complete person with whom we have to deal. He must be separated from his surroundings if he is to be comprehended. If we wish to arrive at the type, we must ascend from the single form to the archetypal form; if we wish to arrive at the human spirit, we must ignore the expressions in which it manifests itself, the special acts which it performs, and observe it in and of itself. We must discover how it behaves in general, not how it has behaved in this or that situation. By comparison, in the case of the type we must separate the universal form from the single forms; in psychology we must separate the single forms only from their surroundings.

Here what applies to organic nature, namely, that we recognize the expression of the archetypal form in the specific being, is no longer valid; here, in perceiving the single forms we recognize the archetypal form itself. The human spiritual being is not one formation of its idea but the formation. When Jacobi believes that, in becoming aware of our inner entity, we at the same time attain the conviction that a unitary being lies at the basis of this entity (intuitive self-apprehension), his thinking is in error because in fact we become aware of this unitary being itself. What in other circumstances is intuition here becomes self-contemplation. With regard to the highest form of being this is also an objective necessity. What the human spirit reads out of phenomena is the highest form of content which it can attain. If the spirit then reflects upon itself, it must recognize itself as the direct manifestation of this highest form — as, indeed, its very bearer. What the spirit finds as unity in the diversity of reality, it must find in its own singleness as immediate existence. What it contrasts with the particular as the general it must attribute to its own individuality as its innate being.

From all this it becomes clear that true psychology can be attained only when we enter into the character of the human spirit in its activity. In place of this method, the attempt has been made nowadays to establish another in which the subject matter of psychology is not the human spirit itself but the phenomena in which the spirit expresses its existence. It is assumed that the external expressions of the spirit can be placed in an external context as can be done with the facts of inorganic nature. In this way the effort is made to establish a 'theory of the soul without the soul'. From our reflections it becomes evident that by such a method we lose sight of the very thing that is important. The spirit should be separated from its manifestations and one should return to the spirit itself as the producer of the latter. Psychologists restrict themselves to the manifestations and lose sight of the spirit. Here, too, people have allowed themselves to be seduced into the erroneous view that the methods of mechanics, physics, etc. should apply to all the sciences

We are able to experience the unity of the soul just as much as its single actions. Every person is conscious of the fact that his thinking, feeling and willing proceed from the ego. Every activity of our personality is bound up with this centre of our being. If we leave this link with the personality out of consideration in any action, it ceases to be a manifestation of the soul. The action then falls under the concept of either inorganic or organic nature. If two balls lie on the table and I push one against the other, the result of that action becomes a physical or physiological occurrence if my purpose and will are left out of consideration. In all manifestations of the spirit—thinking, feeling, willing—the important thing is to recognize these in their essential nature as expressions of the personality. This forms the basis of psychology.

But human beings are not self-contained; they are also part of society. What manifests itself in them is not merely their own individuality but also that of the national grouping to which they belong. What they perform proceeds from the power of the nation as well as from their own power. In their own mission they fulfil something of their national community. The important thing is that their place among their people should be such that the power of their individuality may come to full expression. This is possible only when the national organism is of a type which allows the individual person to find the place where he can exercise some leverage. It must not be left to chance whether or not he finds that place.

The study of the means by which the individual comes to expression within the national community is the subject matter of ethnology and the study of politics and state institutions. The national individuality is the subject of these disciplines. It is their task to show what form the organism of the state must assume if the national individuality is to come to expression within it. The constitution which a people gives to itself must be evolved out of its innermost nature. Here also significant fallacies are being peddled. The study of politics and state institutions is held not to be an experiential science. People believe that the constitution of every nation can be determined according to certain stereotypical patterns.

But the constitution of a nation is nothing more than its individual character brought into fixed forms of law. Anyone who would set out the direction in which a particular activity of a people has to move must not impose upon it anything from outside—he must simply express what lies unconsciously in the character of the people. 'It is not the intelligent person who governs but intelligence; not the rational person, but reason,' says Goethe.

Understanding the reason in national individuality is the method of ethnology. Human beings belong to a whole whose nature consists of an organization based on reason. Here also we can quote a significant saying of Goethe: 'The rational world is to be conceived as a great immortal individuality which unceasingly brings to pass what is necessary and thus makes itself master over the fortuitous.' As psychology investigates the nature of the individual, so the study of politics and state institutions must investigate that 'immortal individuality'.

2. The Social Question

'The Social Question', was published in three instalments in 1898 in Das Magazin für Literatur *(No. 28, July 16, No. 29, July 23, and No. 30, July 30). The article is a review and critique of Dr Ludwig Stein's* The Social Question in the Light of Philosophy *published in 1897. Steiner acknowledges that Stein did an admirable job of assembling the known facts of sociological research but he criticizes Stein's ability to draw proper conclusions from the facts. He proceeds to show how the facts support what Steiner calls the fundamental sociological law. He states that social organizations evolve from units that demand the subjugation of the individual's needs to the needs of the emerging organization. Over time, as the organization matures, the needs of the individual get top priority and the organization becomes a means of allowing the individual maximum opportunity to develop. Steiner calls the goal of sociological development 'anarchistic individualism'.*

To speak about the 'social question' today is not easy. Infinitely much currently contributes to influence our judgement on this question in the most unfavourable way. No subject has been as 'confused by party favour and hatred' as this one. In few areas do the viewpoints stand in such abrupt opposition. What don't they bring up about all this? And how quickly one notices regarding many of these emerging views that they derive from spirits who saunter through the world of facts with the largest possible blinkers on.

But I do not consider the hindrances that party passions place in the way of a desirable assessment of the social question to be the worst. They lead astray only those who stand inside the party machine. One who stands outside the machine always has the possibility of forming a personal opinion. A much more significant hindrance seems to me to be that our thinking minds, our scientifically schooled pillars of culture, never succeed in finding a sure way, a methodological mode, for coming to grips with this question.

Again and again I come to this conviction when I read writings by authors who should be taken altogether seriously on account of their scientific training. I have noticed that in this area the manner of thinking these researchers have acquired under the influence of Darwin has at present had no beneficial effect whatsoever. One must not misunderstand me. I realize that with the Darwinian way of thinking one of the greatest steps forward humanity could take has been achieved. And I do believe that Darwinism must have a beneficial effect when it is properly applied, that is, in accord with its spirit. I myself have produced a book, my *Philosophy of Spiritual Activity*, which, in my opinion, is written entirely in the spirit of Darwinism. In conceiving this book, I had a peculiar experience. I pondered the most intimate questions about human spiritual life. In doing so, I paid no attention at all to Darwinism. And when my thought edifice was finished, it occurred to me: you have here made a contribution to Darwinism.

I discover now that the sociologists in particular do not do this. They enquire of the natural scientists: how do you do it? And then they transfer those methods to their own field. In doing so, they are guilty of a big mistake. They simply carry over natural laws, which hold good for the realm of organic nature, into the area of human spiritual life; exactly the same thing is supposed to hold for human evolution as is observable in that of the animal. Now a sound kernel doubtless does reside in this conception. One surely finds a similar regularity all over the world. But it by no means follows that the same laws therefore apply in all areas. The laws discovered by the Darwinists work in the animal and plant kingdoms. In the human kingdom we have to look for laws that are thought of in the spirit of Darwinism, but that are just as specific to that kingdom as the organic laws of evolution are to the kingdoms named above. We have to seek laws peculiar to the evolution of humanity even though they are to be conceived in the spirit of Darwinism. A simple transfer of the laws of Darwinism onto the evolution of humanity will not be able to lead to satisfying views.

This occurred to me again especially when reading the book that prompted me to write down these thoughts: The Social Question in the Light of Philosophy by Dr Ludwig Stein (Ferdinand Enke Press, Stuttgart, 1897). The approach of the author is completely dominated by the intent to deal with the social question in a way that is in accord with the prevailing view of Darwinistic natural science. 'What Buckle,[31] a human lifetime ago, achieved for the concept of causality in history, namely, that supported by the growing resort to statistics, the unconditional validity of which he proved for historical life altogether, the same thing must happen for evolution after we have mastered the attainments of Darwin and his followers' (page 43). Proceeding in this direction, Stein investigates how the various forms that prevail over the social life of human beings originate. And he seeks to show how 'adaptation' and 'the struggle for existence' play the same role there as in animal evolution. To begin with, I would like to take up one of these forms in order to make his approach plain — that of religion. The human being finds himself in the midst of various natural forces that intervene in his life. They can become useful or harmful to him. They become useful if he finds a means whereby he can use the natural forces in the sense that they serve his existence. Human beings invent tools and equipment in order to render natural forces serviceable. That means they seek to adapt their own existence to that of their environment. Many attempts may be made that prove to be in error. Among infinitely many such, however, there will always be those that hit it right. These remain as the victors; they maintain themselves. The mistaken ones perish. The useful survives the 'struggle for existence'. Among the forces of nature, human beings find the visible accompanied by the invisible. They call them the divine forces alongside the natural. They want to adapt to them, also. They invent religion with the rituals of worship and through this think they can move the divine forces to work for their benefit. Stein considers the origin of marriage, of property, of the state, of language, of law. All these forms arose through the adaptation of the human being to the environment; and the present forms of marriage, property, and so on have lasted because they have proved to be the most useful to the human being.

Thus one can see that Stein is seeking simply to transfer Darwinism to the human realm.

In a subsequent article I will show, by means of the above-named book, where such a transfer leads.

*

In the last issue of this magazine I expressed the view that current assessments of social questions suffer through the way in which thinkers who employ scientific qualifications in this field apply indiscriminately to the [social] development of mankind the results that Darwin and his successors obtained from their studies of the plant and animal kingdoms. I mentioned as one of the books that exemplifies this fault The Social Question by Ludwig Stein.

My opinion about this book is borne out particularly by the fact that Ludwig Stein gathers together the conclusions of modern sociology in a meticulous way, stressing the most important observations arising from this wealth of material. But then he fails to derive from these observations undertaken in the spirit of Darwin any specifically sociological laws, but simply proceeds to interpret the observations by saying that it is possible to discern in them the same laws that govern the animal and plant kingdoms.

Stein has correctly identified the fundamental facts of social evolution. Although he imposes the laws of the 'struggle for survival' and of 'adaptation' on the development of such social institutions as marriage, property, the state, language, law and religion, he discovers in the development of these institutions an important factor that is not to be found in the same measure in the evolution of animals. This factor can be characterized in the following way. All the above-mentioned institutions arise in the first instance in such a way that the interests of the individual recede into the background, while those of the community receive particular emphasis. As a result, these institutions initially take on forms that in the further course of their development have to be counteracted. Marriage, property, the state, and so on could never have developed in the way they did if it had not been for the fact that the tendency of the individual to develop his powers and capacities in an all-round manner had been frustrated. The war of all against all would have prevented any kind of association, for within an association it is always necessary for a person to give up part of his individuality, and man is inclined to do this in the early stages of cultural development.

This is borne out in many ways: for example, there was no such thing as private property in the early stages of human culture. Stein says the following (page 91): 'It is a fact that is confirmed with a degree of unanimity seldom attained by researchers in the field, hence making it all the more convincing, that all property was initially communally owned, remaining such for an immeasurably long period far back into barbarism.' This means that private property, which enables man to assert his individuality, did not exist at the beginning of the [cultural] development of mankind. What better illustration that there was once a time when it was experienced as right to sacrifice the individual to the interests of the community than that during a certain period of time the Spartans used to cast weak individuals out into the wilderness, where they were left to die so that they would not be a burden to the community. Another confirmation can be found in the fact that it did not occur to philosophers of earlier times, such as Aristotle, to regard slavery as barbaric. To Aristotle, for example, it seems quite natural that a certain sector of humankind has to serve another as slaves. One can only hold such a view if one is mainly concerned about the interests of the totality and not about those of the individual. It can easily be demonstrated that the forms of all social institutions at the beginning of cultural evolution were such that the interests of the individual were sacrificed for the sake of the community. However, it is equally true that in the further course of evolution the individual attempts to assert his needs over against those of the community. If we observe closely, a good deal of human history is encompassed in the self-assertion of the individual over against the communities that arose of necessity at the beginning of cultural evolution and that developed at the expense of the individual.

Common sense compels us to acknowledge that social institutions were necessary and that they could only come about through priority being given to common interests. However, it is equally obvious that it is necessary for the individual to resist the sacrifice of his own particular interests. In this way a situation has come about in the course of time, in which social institutions have taken on forms in which the interests of individuals are given more scope than was the case in earlier times. If one rightly understands the nature of our times one might well say that the most advanced members of our society endeavour to develop social forms in such a way that through the forms of human interaction any restrictions on the individual are reduced to a minimum. The idea that a community could be an end in itself is gradually disappearing, and it is seen more and more as providing for the development of the individual. The state, for example, should be constituted in a way that will give the greatest scope to the unrestricted development of the individual. All general arrangements should be made in such a way that they serve the individual rather than the state as such. J.G. Fichte expressed this tendency in an apparently paradoxical yet pertinent way when he said: 'It is the task of the state gradually to make itself redundant.' Underlying this expression is the important truth that initially the individual needs community, for only on the basis of the community can he develop his capacities; however, as soon as these capacities have been developed the tutelage of the community becomes unbearable to him. He then says to himself: I will constitute the community in such a way that it best serves the development of my individual qualities. All state reforms and revolutions in more recent times have asserted the interests of the individual over against those of the community.

It is interesting how Ludwig Stein stresses this fact with regard to every social institution: 'The first social institution, that of marriage, is a process of increasing individualization, complicated by added psychological factors; it is a struggle for individuality' (page 79). Regarding property, Stein says (page 106): 'From a philosophical point of view, the social ideal would be individualism mitigated by the communistic tendency in the state institutions.' Regarding the institution of the state as such, Stein acknowledges 'the obvious tendency within the social process of uninterrupted individualization, leading to the emergence of the individual peak of the sociological pyramid'. When considering the development of language, Stein says: 'Just as sexual communism has moved to individual monogamy, and as communal property has inexorably dissolved into personal property, so the individual wrests his own spiritual personality, his language and his style from that linguistic communism that is bound up with the interests of community. Here, too, is a case of the self-assertion of the individual.' Regarding the development of law, Stein says: 'The law initially encompassed the whole nation, but gradually it took hold of the single physical individuals, and then, within these individuals, of the finest and most delicate psychological ramifications. In this way it presents us with an elusive, yet sufficiently characteristic, picture of the continuing process of the individualization of law' (page 151).

It seems to me that, having stated all these facts, it would have been the task of the sociological philosopher to proceed to describe the fundamental sociological law governing the development of mankind that follows from the above with logical necessity, and that I would like to express as follows: in the early stages of cultural evolution, mankind tends towards the formation of social units; initially the interests of individuals are sacrificed to the interests of those groupings; the further course of development leads to the emancipation of the individual from the interests of the groupings and to the unrestricted development of the needs and capacities of the individual.

Now the point is to draw the logical conclusions from these historical facts. Which social forms can be the only acceptable ones if all social development is tending towards individualization? The answer cannot be too difficult. Any state or society that regards itself as an end in itself has to aim for control over the individual, regardless of the way in which such control is exercised, whether it be in an absolutist, constitutional or republican manner. As soon as the state no longer considers itself an end in itself, but as a means towards an end the principle of state control will no longer be emphasized. All arrangements will be made in such a way that the individual receives the greatest scope. The greatest ideal of the state will be not to control anything. It will be a community that wants nothing for itself, everything for the individual. If one wishes to further developments in this direction, one is bound to oppose everything that tends towards a socialization of social institutions. Ludwig Stein does not do that. He proceeds from the observation of a certain fact, from which he is not able to deduce the right law, to a conclusion that represents a poor compromise between socialism and individualism, between communism and anarchism.

Instead of admitting that we are tending towards individualistic institutions, he tries to lend a hand to a socialistic principle that only admits of individual interests in so far as they do not encroach upon the interests of the community. Regarding the law, for example, Stein says: 'By socialism in the sphere of rights we mean the legal protection of those who are economically weak; the conscious subordination of the interests of the individual to those of a greater common whole, further, to those of the state and eventually to those of the whole of mankind.' Stein regards such a socialization of the law as desirable.

I can account for such a view only by assuming that here a scientist has been so taken in by current slogans that he becomes incapable of drawing the right conclusions from the evidence he presents. The evidence of sociological observation should have forced Stein to represent anarchistic individualism as the social ideal, but for that Stein was not a courageous enough thinker. He seems to know anarchism only in that completely idiotic form in which it is being propagated by bomb-throwing gangs. He confirms what I am saying when he states, for example, on page 597, that 'one can come to an understanding with a working population that is determined, organized and capable of thinking, and for which the laws of logic have binding validity'. The fact is that for someone who knows the laws of social development as Ludwig Stein does, and who can interpret them correctly, which Ludwig Stein is not able to do, it is no longer possible to come to an understanding with workers whose thoughts have been shaped by communist ideology.

Ludwig Stein is a great scholar. His book proves this. Ludwig Stein is also a naive sociologist. His book proves this. Both are apparently quite compatible in our time. We have attained a high level of development in the sphere of pure observation. But a good observer is far from being a good thinker. And Ludwig Stein is a good observer. What he can tell us as a result of his own and other people's observations is important for us; the conclusions he draws from these observations are irrelevant.

I have read his book with interest. It was very useful for me. I have learned much from it. However, I was always compelled to draw different conclusions from the data presented. Where he allows the facts to speak through him, I find him stimulating; where he speaks himself, I am bound to oppose him.

Yet I have to ask myself: how is it that Ludwig Stein, in spite of his true insights, arrives at the wrong social ideals? And here I come back to my original statement: he is incapable of really deriving social laws from social facts. Had he been able to do this he could never have arrived at such a poor compromise between socialism and anarchism. Anyone who is really capable of recognizing certain laws could not fail to act accordingly.

I have to come back again and again to the fact that the thinkers in our age are cowards. They do not have the courage to draw the appropriate conclusions from their observations. They are prepared to compromise with the illogical. It would be far better if they did not touch the social question at all. It is far too important. This question does not exist simply to provide someone with the opportunity to draw a few trivial conclusions, worthy of a moderate social reformer, from fairly solid observations; to give a few lectures on the subject; and then to publish them in book form. I regard Stein's book as a demonstration of what our scholars are really capable of, yet also of how incapable they are of actual thinking. What we need at the present time is courage; the courage to think, the courage to be consistent; but alas, we only have cowardly thinkers.

I would go so as far as to say that faint-heartedness in thinking has been the outstanding characteristic of our age. To blunt the consequences arising from a thought and to juxtapose another 'equally valid' one — that is a general tendency today. Stein recognizes that human development is tending towards individualism. However, he lacks the courage to consider how we can move from the present conditions to a social order that can give scope to this individualism. E. Munsterberg recently translated a book by Brussels professor Adolf Prins (Freedom and Social Duty by Adolf Prins, authorized translation by E. Munsterberg, Otto Leibman Press, Berlin, 1897). Prins is fully aware of those facts whose implications would sweep away both socialism and communism in an instant: 'And I think that among those elements that form the eternal foundation of mankind, the heterogeneity of the human being is one of the most persistent.' No socialist or communist form of government or social order is capable of taking adequate account of the natural diversity of human beings. Any organization that is in any way pre-determined in its nature by any principles must of necessity suppress the full and unhindered development of the individual in order to maintain its own integrity as an organism. Even a sociologist who in principle acknowledges the full development of all individuals as justified will, in the course of the practical realization of his ideals, seek to eliminate those individual idiosyn-crasies that do not happen to fit into his programme.

The train of thought of this Belgian professor is inter-esting. He admits right from the beginning that any accumulation of power in one place is harmful. He therefore supports those medieval institutions with their

legal and administrative systems based on local associations and regional individualities over against the tendency, derived from the Romans, to centralize power,
neglecting any individual or regional peculiarities (page
40ff.). Prins even opposes the system of universal suffrage
because he feels that a minority might be oppressed by
what might be an insignificant majority. Yet he too sug-
gests unwholesome compromises between socialism and
individualism. From all his considerations, it should have
been clear to this professor that all welfare and prosperity
arise from the activity of individuals. He does not have the
courage to admit this and says: 'But the greatest degree of
individuality does not arise from excessive individualism'
(page 63). I would like to reply to this: it is impossible to
speak of 'excessive' individualism, for nobody can tell
how much of an individual's capacities and gifts are lost
when they are prevented from unfolding freely. He who
wishes to apply moderation in this sphere can never know
which slumbering capacities he might be eradicating from
the world by his clumsy measures. This is not the place for
making practical suggestions. However, this is the place to
say that he who can read the development of mankind
rightly can only support a social order that has as its aim
the unrestricted, all-around development of individuals,
and that abhors the domination of any one person by
another. The question that then remains is how each
individual is to cope with himself. Each individual will
solve this problem for himself if all sorts of communities
do not get in the way.

The worst of all forms of government is that propagated by the social democrats. They want to get out of the frying pan by jumping into the fire. We have to accept the fact that social democracy is one of the ghosts walking around in our time. And since, as everyone knows, red is the most exciting colour, it has a terrible effect on many people — but only on those who cannot think. Those who can think know that the realization of the ideals of social democracy would mean the suppression of all individuality. However, because it is impossible to suppress — for human evolution has set its sight on human individuality once and for all — the victory of social democracy would at the same time be its downfall.

Those who are overawed by the tattered red flag of social democracy to such an extent that they believe that every theory about social life must be lubricated with the necessary drop of social oil cannot see that. This is how oily they are, the Ludwig Steins and the Adolf Prinses.

Both do not quite know what to do. They think. This activity ought to be turning them into individualists or, to put it bluntly, into theoretical anarchists. But they are afraid; in fact, they are absolutely terrified by the implications of their own thinking, and therefore they dress it a little with the oil of Bismarck's state socialism and with the social democratic nonsense of Messrs Marx, Engels and Liebknecht. He who has many things to offer will please some!

However, this does not apply to thinkers! In my view, everyone should stand up wholeheartedly for his own convictions with all their implications and consequences. There is nothing to lose. Should they turn out be wrong, then another one is bound to win anyway. The question whether our views will win the day we must leave to the future to decide. All we should be concerned about is to stand firm in the struggle.

People who specialize in thinking should definitely be involved in the discussion about the social question for they are known for the fact that their discipline does not allow them to become swayed by party passions. However, even thinkers need to be passionate in one respect — they need to stand ruthlessly by their own views. The thinkers of our time lack this kind of ruthlessness.

In the introduction to his book, Ludwig Stein laments the fact that the philosophers of the day pay so little attention to the social question. I cannot go along with him in this. I could only agree with Stein if our philosophers were thinkers with the courage of their convictions. But as things stand at the moment, nothing spectacular could come from the participation of our philosophers in the discussion on the social question. Ludwig Stein's book bears this out to me. In it he says nothing of any possible relevance to the question. He serves up the same old stew that we get from all the middle-of-the-road parties and candidates-of-compromise of all nations, dressed with a bit of philosophical salad, not thereby making it any more palatable.

3. The Social Question and Theosophy

'The Social Question and Theosophy',[32] is the text of a lecture Steiner gave on 26 October 1905. In content it closely parallels an essay he wrote at about the same time, published in English under the title 'The Science of the Spirit and the Social Question'. This latter has been published several times in English and is well known as the place where Steiner first stated what he considered a fundamental social law. The lecture was chosen as it is less widely known and because it includes a very interesting example that illustrates how Steiner hoped people would experiment with his fundamental social law. Specifically, he makes the radical suggestion that a group of people wishing to free itself from the negative effects of capital form a community in which each member placed his earnings in a common account and that all live from this account. In this fashion a person would free his or her self from the necessity, otherwise present in modern society, of having to work for his or her own welfare. This suggestion has been implemented to varying degrees in different anthroposophical communities, notably the Camphill Communities and the Rudolf Steiner Fellowship Community. It was also behind the experiment known as an 'income community' conducted by the late Ernst Barkhoff and his co-workers in connection with the founding of the first anthroposophical bank in Bochum, Germany.

The social question, which is to occupy us today, did not, as will immediately become clear for everyone, arise out of a mere idea or out of the undoubted need of a few people, but is a question that confronts us with facts as strongly and clearly today as ever. Anyone who looks around just a little in the surrounding world will know what a distinct language these facts speak. It could well be that someone who does not want to hear this language of the facts will find out in the not too distant future that he has closed his ears too long to what was necessarily going on. With regard to the social question, the human being of the present is standing within the conflict that is at times still playing itself out under the surface of our social order. Anyone who wants to say, more or less precisely, how the social conflict has increased in extent and violence does not need to go any further into externals; he needs only to draw attention to the violent workers' movement on the occasion of the work stoppage at Crimmitschau, to the miners' strike on the occasion of the lockout of the elec-trical workers, and, in sum, to what is going on in Eastern Europe.[33] In all this we will discern the social question being lived out.

The reproach has often been addressed to theosophy that it has a number of dreamers among its followers, that it seeks to work only in those areas to which one retreats from the great common questions of the time, where one wants to linger in leisurely contemplation of the human soul. And so they say: theosophists are a few people who have nothing particular to do, who in an egoistical way want to retreat into the self and cultivate it in the manner of theosophy. It is easy to reproach theosophy that it wants to stand apart from the great conflict of the day, from what affects humanity in the present time. Theosophists should be doing something about that. They should keep pointing out that theosophists must be wherever there is something to investigate and reflect on regarding warranted human affairs in the present, they must have a clear heart and clear thinking, they must not lose themselves in some cloudy Utopia, but rather must stand within everyday affairs, helping and caring. And this other reproach can also easily be made—that theosophy is touted as a universal cure for all the evils and grievances of the present. That also is not so. To be sure, it is claimed that theosophy, the theosophical movement, has something to do with all that and must prepare itself in the present for a better future, but not in the sense of rulership, not as a universal cure do we extol theosophy; rather, we only want to show that with it something so comprehensive is given that without it today we cannot progress in the most essential things that we should be concerned about, and that all speculation and reforms must remain half-baked unless the human being approaches the matter from a theosophical perspective. The doctrines of thinkers about grand encompassing cosmic connections, about the universal law of world destiny and world events occupy us in the inner circles of our theosophical movement not merely so we can gaze at the starry vastness at leisure, but rather because we know that these laws we are studying and which are active in the great cosmos are also active in the human heart, in the soul, and in fact give the soul the capacity really to see into the life of the immediate present.

We are sort of like an engineer who absorbs himself for years in his technical studies, but not in order to engage in contemplations of the mysteries of the calculus and marvel at them; rather we seek the laws which we then apply to human life, as the engineer builds bridges and applies the laws to reality.

There is also something here that is universal and widespread and opens up a further horizon. Who would dare to present thinking as a universal remedy, even though this thinking is necessary for what can happen in the cosmos? Theosophy is no dead matter, no dead theory. No, it is something life-awakening. It is not a matter of the concepts, the ideas, that we take on. What is told here does not have the intention of dealing with the ideas as such, nor the intention of developing interesting notions about hidden facts, but rather, what is here passed before the human soul has a very special quality. Non-theosophists may believe it or not, but anyone who has occupied himself with it knows that what I am about to say is correct in practice. Anyone who has applied himself to how, in theosophy, the world and life are considered will notice his life of the senses and of soul becoming something different from what they were before. He learns to think in another way and will observe human circumstances in a more unbiased way than previously.

We have a distant future in mind when we speak of

awakening higher powers through inner development. But for the immediate future we also keep an eye on the life that we can bring about through theosophical development—that is, the possibility of coming to a comprehensive, clear and unbiased assessment of the human situations immediately surrounding us. Our culture, with all the scientific character which it has developed up to now, has come up with theories that are impotent regarding life. The theosophical world-view will not produce such impotent theories. It will teach mankind thinking, awaken thinking forces in mankind that are not powerless regarding realty, but will empower us to take hold of human evolution itself, to take hold of the immediate conduct of life.

Let me introduce a small symptomatic example that will further clarify what I mean to say. Recently a clear example in the political field was provided by a Prussian government councillor who went on leave to find work in America, to take part in and get to know conditions there.[34] A state councillor is normally called upon to be active in human evolution. Taken in a higher sense, it is his duty and obligation to let something live in his heart that corresponds to real conditions and not merely to theories. And if he has nothing that chimes with the conditions, then his theory is impotent. This man, who for years previously had been called upon to deal with the human element, got to know the human element himself. Of course what I am saying entails not the least reproach against the individual man. This deed is to the highest degree honourable and bold, as well as admirable. But what he has written is a symptom of what is at stake. It shows the discrepancy in his orientation towards the world and towards workers. Here are just a few words from his book As a Worker in America [4th edition, Berlin 1905, p. 31][35]: 'How often when I previously saw a healthy man begging did I ask with moral indignation why doesn't the lout go to work? Now I knew why. In theory things look different from practice; even the most unappetizing aspects of the national economy are easy enough to handle at your desk.'

There is no greater mark of poverty than when someone who is called upon to take action says that the theory which he had does not agree with the conditions. Here is the point at which one can take hold of the matter; just as logic enables people to think at all, and just as no one can become a mathematician without manipulating logic, just so no one can develop the power of practical thinking without theosophy. Look at the national economy that is overwhelming our developmental [free] market. If you set about looking into things with healthy, comprehensive thinking, theosophical thinking, you will find that things that are supposed to be guideposts, emanating perhaps from university professors or party leaders, are dry theory suitable for being dealt with at a desk, but useless when one is facing reality. Such things reveal themselves, for instance, at congresses. One just has to observe more closely. Congresses in general bear this character. If those who busy themselves would care to descend into practical life, they would soon find that they are capable of nothing. Merely gazing at life does not do it. Nor can someone who judges from the standpoint of today's customary culture pass judgment on the women's question or the social question, nor can someone judge who merely looks at things, for nothing is achieved by that either.

Now if you were to ask the gentleman who wrote these words what can lead to an improvement, then you would find that he has only learned how it looks; but how things should be done, that is a different question altogether. It is also not a question that can be answered in an hour or a day. It cannot be answered at all by theoretical debate. No theosophist worthy of the name will say to you: I have this programme for the social question, or the women's question, for the vivisection question, or about the care of animals and so forth. On the contrary, he will say: put people who are theosophists into the institutions dealing with all these questions, set such people in professorial chairs for economics; then they will have the ability to develop the thinking which will lead to making the individual branches of their activity into guideposts in the realm of public life. As long as this is not the case, people in this realm will be charlatans and will have to witness the world collapsing around them, and how idle verbosity in congresses shows itself in its uselessness.

I say this not out of fanaticism, but rather on the basis of what in every theosophist is a real theosophical attitude, real theosophical thinking. Theosophical thinking develops clarity about the various realms of life, a clear, objective view of the forces and powers working in the world. To look at the matter rightly, that is what theosophical life enables you to do. Therefore theosophy is not a panacea in the ordinary sense, rather it is the foundation of contemporary life.

After these introductory words, let us give a few indications on the basis of the facts about what has given the social question its special stamp. Whoever wants to see what will happen must know the laws of development, may not have dry theories but must know the laws of the development of humanity. We cannot find these laws through some sort of abstract science. Theosophy does not proceed abstractly. It proceeds from clear contemplative thinking. And so let me indicate with at least a few words how the life of today has shaped itself, how this life today has come to be. One who looks more closely at life will realize that some self-knowledge also belongs in these realms in order to see clearly. First I will picture the outer facts, then I will say a few things concerning what it is actually all about.

Every one of us knows what the human being needs in order to live. We all have an idea of what food and clothing we need. A few figures will tell us how much the majority has of all these things. All we need to do in this regard is to examine the tax structure. It has been told repeatedly, but we can bring it to mind again. In Prussia, someone who has an income of less than 900 marks pays no taxes. One can very easily check how many people in Prussia have an income of less than 800 or 900 marks. That is 21 million people. Ninety-five per cent of the total population have less than 3000 marks income. Take England. Only those who have an income over 150 pounds are taxed. [...] You see, we have plenty of figures which indicate the number of people who have what is required as basic necessities.

Look at statistics. They speak a distinct language. But what does that have to do with our self-knowledge? A lot. For it is a matter of gaining the right standpoint for ourselves regarding these facts. And in this connection people let themselves miss out a great deal on what is right. What are people around us doing? What is the cause of their receiving this low income? It is what we give them for what they do for us. We now make no distinction between workers and non-workers, between proletariat and non-proletariat. For if one makes this distinction, then the matter is already entirely false. And that is the mistake of all our national economic considerations, that one does not proceed from self-knowledge, but rather from theory.

[The following sentences of the transcript reveal a few discrepancies, so that the original wording cannot be reconstructed. By the gist of it, Rudolf Steiner most likely described how every person lives from the products that another has produced. Products are produced even for someone out of work whose means or livelihood are insufficient. Even the seamstress working for starvation wages wears clothes that have been produced in turn for a starvation wage. Compare the paragraphs written in the same year in the essay 'Spiritual Science and the Social Question', in *Lucifer Gnosis*.]

And if in our emotions and perceptions we are able to feel a certain pain over the fact that the clothes we have on have been produced for a starvation wage, then we are looking deep into the heart of the question. When in all this you think about what you wear in the way of clothing, what you put in your mouth for nourishment, where it comes from, only then will you grasp the social question in all its depth. Not through speculation, but rather through a living contemplation does one get an insight into what it is all about.

It is not right when it is said that today's misery, even if we could portray it in its direst colours, is greater than it was in former centuries. That is not the case. We would be committing real falsification of objective reality. Just try to study conditions objectively in the city of Cologne today and 120 years ago, and you will see that much has got better. And even so we are faced with the social question. We are faced with it because human beings have gone through yet another evolution, and this is because in large measure they have come to thinking, to self-consciousness, and because their needs have greatly changed. If we study the question thus, we are indeed of necessity directed towards the broad contexts that arise for us in world history if we are not, like modern researchers, too short-sighted. In order to judge these things it is necessary to get to know the great laws of life. What has caused social affairs to take this shape? It is the manner and method which the human spirit has assumed. Look back to the time of the French Revolution. At that time other things were demanded. It was a tendency more towards the juridical that brought out the ideal of Liberty — Equality — Fraternity. The French revolutionary heroes in Western Europe called for liberty. Those now battling in Eastern Europe call for bread. It is simply two sides of the same coin, two different demands of human beings who have learned to put such questions because their souls have undergone a transformation.

We have to study this transformation of the soul more closely. We must study and understand why these demands have arisen in the souls of the great masses of human beings today — and they will continue to grow in the course of the centuries. At this point the theosophical world conception comes in with practical application, underpinning our comprehension. Only someone who understands the case is qualified to judge it. The only person who is able to look into souls is the person who, in the great world context, sees what is going on in these souls. And only someone who understands something of the laws of the soul is able to effect something in souls and lead into the future.

As a small aside, the sciences of today, biology, Darwinism, Haeckelianism,[36] have brought us great ideas. So also the idea that each living entity, in the first stages of its existence, even in its germinal state, recapitulates the forms of life that have previously been gone through out in nature. This brief recapitulation of the various stages occurs also in that being which includes them all, climbing higher on the ladder of evolution than all others: the human being. Assume that a spirit had consciousness at a time before there were any human beings, then he would have had to know not only what had already happened, but he would also—by contrast—have had to form a picture of future evolution. He would have had to form a picture for the future out of the animal condition of that time. Only the human being, who in his germinal configuration recapitulates the preceding conditions, can show us what to do. It is the doing that must pass beyond all knowing. No knowing occupies itself with anything but what was. But if we want to work into the future, we have to do things that haven't been there yet. The great laws that are to be realized in the future show us this. In a certain way everything that is to come about in the future has already been there in the past, namely, through intuition. A spirit who had intervened at that time would have had to have had intuition in order to be able to find out about the hidden laws of existence that apply to the past and the future. That is why theosophy cultivates intuition. That is what reaches out beyond the mere physical experience of the world. Theosophy looks for the laws that are to be cognized by intuition and which lead us into the future of the human race.[37]

One of these great world laws that can be a guide for us is the law of reincarnation. First, it renders understandable for us how in higher spiritual realms what applies as law is nothing other than what Darwin and Haeckel have intimated. It renders comprehensible why this or that was felt as a need in any given age. Anyone who immerses himself in these things knows the last time in which there was life thirsting for universal freedom, when human beings took up impulses for which they should be calling today. The ones who today call for liberty and equality—I say this with the same objective certainty with which natural scientists speak about the physical—all those souls who today cry for liberty and equality have learned it at another stage of their existence, in an earlier incarnation. The greatest needs of the human being of today were embodied in the early time of Christianity, in the first Christian centuries. All human beings have taken up this push for equality which faces human beings today in spiritual life. Christianity brought the message of equality before God. In times prior to that, there had been no such equality.

I do not say what I have just said in a derogatory way, I say it with the same sober objectivity with which I would speak of any scientific problem. If one considers the soul as such and then everything which creates outward inequalities, the same soul that once assimilated the impulse 'they are equal before God and before human-kind' finds that everything that determines outward inequality has no meaning for contemporary life. When the grave closes over us we will all be and become equal. What the soul has taken up lives on in the soul and emerges in a different form. If we consider cultural progress from the perspective of the macrocosm we come to tremendous implications regarding education. I have already drawn attention to what this pedagogy on earth was like in pre-Christian times. Let us look back into Egyptian times. A large number of people there were occupied with work, the difficulty of which a man of today can no longer estimate. They laboured willingly. And why? Because they knew that this life is one among many. Each one said to himself: the one who is in charge of my work is like the person I will be sometime. This life must be compensated in different incarnations, for it directs itself out of this knowledge.

Linked with this is the law of karma. What I have experienced in one life is either deserved or will be compensated for in later times. If it had merely gone on like that, however, then the human being would have overlooked the kingdom of the earth. This one life would not have been important to him. In that regard Christianity took educational measures in order to have this life between birth and death be of importance to him. It is merely illusory when Christianity deviates from that, for it has pointed strongly to the beyond; it has even made eternal punishment and eternal bliss a function of a single life.

Whoever believes that the one life is of primary importance learns to take this life seriously. It pivots around the truths that are suitable for the human being, and it is suitable for the human being to be raised in the idea of this one earth life. Such were the two tasks: education regarding the importance of earthly life between birth and death, and, on the other hand, that outside this earthly life everyone is equal before God. This earthly life has been bearable only by being so considered that all are equal before God. Whoever looks at it that way will observe a descent into the physical world in the development of mankind since the rise of Christianity. More and more the human being feels committed to physical existence. Through this he transferred the importance of the rule of the equality before God more and more to equality in material existence itself.

That picture should not be misunderstood. The soul that 1800 years ago was accustomed to claiming equality for the beyond now brings the impulse for equality with it, but in connection with what is important today — 'equality before Mammon'. Please do not see a criticism or anything pejorative in this, rather the objective confirmation of a cosmic law of the developing soul. One must study the course of time this way. Then one will understand that only one thing will again bring about in this soul a change in direction, an ascent, namely, if we get the soul who is calling for equality back into the beyond. Towards the beyond we looked up, from the here-and-now we looked out. Today, due to this impulse, the soul is turned back upon itself. Today it seeks the same thing in the here-and-now. If it is to find an ascent again, it must find the spirit in the present, the inwardness, in the soul element itself. That is what the theosophical world movement is striving for: to prepare the soul for the third stage,[38] because it is filled with God, filled with divine wisdom, and will thereby again know how to place itself in the world, so that it will again find the harmony between itself and the surrounding world.

Such thoughts have value in giving direction. We cannot bring this about from one day to the next. But we also cannot consider our individual deeds alone. Every deed must stand under some influence. Then it becomes practical, then it is something, then it is no dry theory but rather immediate life because we are looking into the workings of the soul.

Our national economists and our social theorists today so often say: the human being is only the product of outer circumstances. A person has become what he is because he has lived in a particular set of external conditions. That is what social democracy seriously argues, for example, saying that the human being becomes what the environment makes of him. Because due to the entire development of industry he has become a proletarian worker, he has also become one in his soul, the way he has evolved through just these conditions. The human being is a product of circumstances. We can often hear that. Let us study the conditions themselves, let us consider what is round about us, what we are most dependent on. Are we dependent merely on nature? No! We notice what we are dependent on only when we stand starving in front of the bakery and have nothing in our pockets to buy anything with.

All these conditions are made and put into effect by other human beings. The spirit that is evolving through history has brought these conditions about. People have created today's conditions out of concern for their own welfare, sometimes only a short time before. Thus anyone who thinks people are dependent on circumstances is reasoning in a circle because the circumstances were brought about by people. If we picture this to ourselves we must say that it is not a matter of the circumstances, rather we have to look at how the circumstances have come to be. It is idle to insist on saying: the human being is dependent on his circumstances. In 50 years the human being will also be dependent on the conditions that surround him. You can concede to every social democrat[39] that the human being is dependent on circumstances, but on those that we cause today, that emanate from our disposition, from our soul. We create the social conditions! And what will live then will be the crystallized perceptions and feelings that we put out into the world today.

This shows us what it is all about — that one must learn the laws under which the world is evolving. It cannot be a matter of science; rather, it can only be an intuition of what we must contribute as law. This comes directly out of a perception that seems very fantastic to most people, but which is much clearer and more objective than much of the fantastic imagination of our scientists; a perception that can tell what lives in the soul and then crystallizes outwardly can also, out of the wisdom, out of the divine in the soul tell what an individual can spread out into the world and what is proper for humanity.

If in the future you want to be surrounded by such

circumstances, if you want to have things organized that way as an institution which will satisfy people, about which people will be able to say, 'That's it—we want to live under these conditions,' then you must first pour humanity into these conditions, so that humanity will stream out of them again. The deepest humanity, the deepest inwardness of soul must first stream out of our own hearts into the world. Then the world will be an image of the soul, and in the soul there will be an image of the world. This will be able to satisfy people again. Therefore human beings cannot expect anything from all those quackeries in the social area that are perpetrated by looking at outer circumstances. These outer circumstances are made by human beings; they are nothing other than human souls which have streamed outwards. The first things that have to be worked with, what needs to be taken up first as the social question, are the souls of today which produce the environment of tomorrow. You can see how better conditions stream into the environment if only you would study it. Again and again I hear politicians dealing with social affairs say: make the conditions better and human beings will become better. Just let these people study what individual sects pursue as soul culture, developing themselves cut off from world evolution, just let them study what the latter contribute to the shaping of outer conditions. If human beings realize that the improvement of conditions depends on themselves, if they acquire theosophical knowledge, and if they recognize the first fundamental principle to establish the kernel of a universal brotherhood[40] and develop it in themselves as a social feeling for the surrounding world, then real social development is possible, and one is prepared for what will happen in the near future. Our entire national economy today lives under false premises. Therefore our theories are mostly false because they proceed from assumptions entirely different from those that arise out of the human being and from humanity. One starts with production, or one believes one can achieve something with the development of compensation. All thinking moves in this direction. To be sure, an improvement will not occur immediately with a change in thinking. But it will occur when the direction is changed. Moreover, our proletariat has no inkling about what the issue is here. What it demands is more pay and shorter hours. Take a look at the worker in any particular sector, say the electricity industry, which has been unionized in order through this collective to get better pay and working conditions. What does he want with these better working conditions? He wants a different relation regarding compensation to be established between him and his employer.

That is all he wants. The conditions of production do not change. All that happens is that the worker gets higher wages [...]. That is all that happens. It is just a shift in capital.

But that doesn't really change anything much at all, because if one gets more pay today, food will be more expensive tomorrow. It is not possible to bring about any

kind of improvement for the future in this way. This
ongoing endeavour is based on false thinking. There it is a
matter of production and consumption. Here a great
comprehensive worldwide law about work applies. One
has to know this. Certain people who are used to thinking
in today's national economic terms will say perhaps that I
am obscuring things. One who has worked his way
through to theosophy has, as a rule, gone through today's
thinking. Theosophy should be active in us as a life
impulse. But just as every thought will enter into us and
stimulate every action in us, so this also should stimulate
us. We need not think that we can realize it right away.
Also, the government councillor who does not live in dry
theories can look at life entirely differently. He does not
need to travel to America in order to get the idea that
someone who does not have any work is not necessarily a
lazy lout. In the course of time work has greatly changed
its form.

Take a look at ancient Greece. What was work in those
days? The worker stood in an entirely different relation to
his master. At that time work was slavery. The worker
could be compelled by force to work. What he received
from his master was his living. But his master took the
proceeds of the work; it had nothing whatever to do with
the particular relation of the worker to his master—he had
to work. Moreover, he was maintained under precarious
conditions; he was not compensated for the things he did.
There we have labour under duress, without pay.

[A] commodity is the result of something other than

directly compensated work. Thus its value also has nothing to do with what is paid as wages. Look at today's situation. Today we have jobs for which workers are partly compensated — partly. What they bring in flows as profit into the pockets of the entrepreneur. Thus work is partly compensated. What does this make the worker himself? He invests his labour power in this work. In Greece, when one was confronting a unit of work, it was a product of slavery. Today's commodity involves something entirely different. Today the luxury that I receive is crystallized labour for which the worker is compensated. If we reflect on this, we will find that a half-freedom has taken over from the old slavery. A contractual relationship has taken its place. In that way labour has become a commodity in the shape of the labourer. So we have labour that is half compelled and half voluntary. And the course of evolution is in the direction of completely voluntary work. This path no one will change or reject. Just as the Greek labourer did his work under the compulsion of his master and a present labourer works under the compulsion of wages, similarly in the future only freedom will obtain. Labour and compensation will in future be completely separated.

That will constitute the health of social conditions in the future. You can see it already today. Work will be a voluntary performance out of the recognition of necessity, out of the realization that it must be done. People perform it because they look at the person and see that he needs work done for him. What was labour in antiquity? It was tribute, it was performed because it had to be performed. And what is the labour of the present time? It is based on self-interest, on the compulsion that egoism exerts on us. Because we want to exist, we want labour to be paid for. We work for our own sake, for the sake of our pay. In the future we will work for our fellow human beings, because they need what we can provide. That is what we will work for. We will clothe our fellow human beings, we will give them what they need — in completely free activity. Compensation must be completely separated from this. Labour in the past was tribute, in the future it will be sacrifice. It has nothing to do with self-interest, nothing to do with compensation. If I base my labour on consumer demand with regard to what humanity needs, I stand in a free relation to labour and my work is a sacrifice for humanity. Then I will work with all my powers, because I love humanity and want to place my capacities at its disposal.

That has to be possible, and is possible only when one's livelihood is separated from one's labour. And that is going to happen in the future. No one will be the owner of the products of labour. People must be educated for voluntary work, one for all and all for one. Everyone has to act accordingly. If you were to found a small community today in which everyone throws all their income into a common bank account and everyone works at whatever they can do, then one's livelihood is not dependent on what work one can do, but rather this livelihood is effected out of the common consumption. This brings about a greater freedom than the coordination of pay with production does. If that happens, we will gain a direction which corresponds to needs. Even today, this can flow into every law, every decree. Of course, not absolutely, but approximately. Even today one can organize factories in the right way. But that demands healthy, clear, sober thinking in the spirit of theosophy. If such things penetrate into human souls, then something will be able to live again in these human souls. And just as the one determines the other, so this life of the human soul will also determine that the outer arrangements will be a mirror image of it, so that our labour will be a sacrificial offering and no longer self-interest — so that what controls the relationship with the outer world is not compensation, but rather what is in us. We offer to humanity what we have in our power to do. If we cannot do much, then we cannot offer much; if we have a lot, then we offer a lot.

We must know that every activity is a cause of endless effects and that we may allow nothing that is in our soul to go unused. We will be making every offering out of our soul if we completely renounce any pay that can accrue to us from external circumstances, if we do so not for our own sake, not for the sake of our welfare, but rather for the sake of necessity. We want to strengthen the soul through the law of its own inner being, so that it learns to place its powers at the disposal of the whole from points of view other than the law of wages and self-interest. There have been thinkers who in some contexts have already thought in this way. In the first half of the nineteenth century there have been thinkers who referred to such a feature of a grand, soul-based contemplation of cosmic law. Is this feature not a sanctification of labour? Are we not able to lay it on the altar of humanity? Thus labour becomes anything but a burden. It becomes something into which we place what is most sacred for us, our compassion for humanity, and then we can say: labour is sacred because it is a sacrifice for humankind.

Now there have been people who in the first half of the nineteenth century spoke of 'sacred industry'. Saint-Simon[41] was one of those who had an inkling of the great ideas of the future. Anyone who studies his writings will, if they are deepened in a theosophical sense, gain a great deal for our time. Saint-Simon referred in a basic way to a type of living together as in an association. He proposed associations into which the single individuals deposited tribute, making their livelihood independent. He had great ideas about the development of humanity, and discovered several things. He said that the human races corresponded to a planned development, and souls made their appearance one after another and worked their way upwards. That is the way to regard the development of humanity, for that leads to the correct view. He also spoke of a planetary spirit that changes itself into other planets on which humanity will live. In short, here is an economist whose works you can read and who lived in the first half of the nineteenth century. You read his work like a theosophical book.

Today the palingenesis [continued rebirth, metempsychosis] of soul existence can be proved. Whoever acknowledges Haeckel will also have to acknowledge reincarnation if Haeckel's ideas are carried further. Fourier[42] also thought in this way. You can find in him a primitive theosophy. Thus theosophy's first major principle for our social life—to establish the kernel of a universal brotherhood—is the only thing that can propagate healthy conditions in the context in which we live for anyone who looks at things the way they are. This view of the theosophists is not impractical. On the contrary, it is more practical than the view of all those social theorists (you will have to admit this if you apply these theories to life), and only someone like the latter will say with good old Kolb: studying theories of national economy is no burden. Only if theosophy comes to be heard in debates on the social question can a healthy way of looking at it, a healthy thinking come into it. So it is necessary for someone who wants to see and hear in this area to come to terms with theosophy.

For theosophists two things are clear, not out of fanaticism but rather out of a knowledge that comes from looking at life: it is possible to stick with dry theory and relegate the matter to people who will later have to admit that at the desk it looks different from what it turns out to be in life out there. Then one will have to wait a long time, and what must come will come anyway. In the end, living theory will have to intervene in life. One can hear it already today—already today one can argue about what theosophy has to say about the social question. Then it is not enough to hear just one lecture; rather one has to deal with theosophy in its entirety. From it one will derive the gift, the ability, in a healthy way to view life from top to bottom in its most secret and intimate forces, then healing and blessing can soon come into our social order.

Let us bring about what should happen as much as we can in ourselves. The reshaping of labour, not working for pay, is a sacrifice. Then we will have done our duty, then we will have regarded life in a healthy way. Or else we will keep looking at the world with dry theories alien to life. Then it could turn out that future humanity might say: Questions were raised; when these questions were there to be raised, when recovery in a good way was possible, that was just when they did not want to study them. Goethe once said: 'Revolutions are entirely impossible if the rulers do their duty.'[43] He knew who was to blame for revolution. Let us try to consider what the history of the future will say about our present. You have seen what time has wrought, until the earth was drenched with blood, and how the time has raised the most burning questions in an even more frightful way.

4. Memoranda of 1917

The memoranda of 1917 are presented here for the first time in English.[44] They are real historical documents that found their way into the hands of leading Central European statesmen in 1918. The history of the memoranda is discussed in the introduction to this volume.

Among the reasons they give for having to continue the war, the spokesmen for the Entente argue that Germany attacked them. They thus assert that they must bring Germany into such a condition of powerlessness that henceforth any possibility of Germany executing another attack is removed. All other causes of the war are submerged in this moral indictment against Germany.

Given this indictment, Germany is blocked from expressing in a completely unvarnished way how it was driven to war. In place of that, there are at the moment only doctrinaire statements about the cause of the war that sound like the conclusions of a professor who is not telling what he has seen but, rather, who explains from documents what he has discovered about distant happenings. The comments of the German Chancellor about the events surrounding the outbreak of war are of a similar character. These statements are unfit to make an impression. They are simply rejected by opposing them with other unjustified or, indeed, justified statements.

On the other hand, if the facts were to be simply narrated, the following would result:

1. In the summer of 1914, Germany was not prepared to take the initiative for war.

2. Austria-Hungary had for a long time been placed in the necessity of doing something to counter the threatening danger of Austro-Hungarian territory being reduced in the southern part as a result of the union of the southern Slavs under the leadership of the Serbians outside of Austria. One can easily concede that the murder of Archduke Franz Ferdinand and the whole business of the ultimatum was only an excuse for Austria-Hungary. If this excuse had not been used, then it would have been another one. Austria could not have remained Austria without doing something about the security of its southeast provinces, or solving the Slav problem by means of generous alternative action. But Austrian politics had bled to death on the question of alternative action since 1879. Better stated, Austrian politics bled to death because such alternative action could not be found. There was a failure to master the Slav question. To the extent that Austria-Hungary must be considered as the cause of war — and thus Germany, too, because it could not abandon Austria-Hungary without having to fear that in a few years it would face the Entente without Austria as an ally — to this extent it must be recognized that the Slav question

contains the reason which provoked war. The 'alternative action' is thus the international solution of the Slav question. This international solution was demanded of Austria, not of Russia. For Russia will always be able to throw its fundamental Slav character into the scales of the solution. The Austro-Hungarians can oppose the weight of the Russian influence only with the weight of the liberation of the west Slavs. Such liberation can only proceed from the point of view of making autonomous all branches of national life in relation to national existence and all that is connected with it. One simply must not shrink from complete freedom in the sense of making autonomous or federalizing the life of the nation. Such federalization already exists in the federal structures of the German state which in a certain sense is the historically prepared model for that which must be developed in Central Europe up to a fully federalized free form of all those situations of life which have their impulses in the human being himself — thus not dependent directly, like the military-political realm, on geographical relations and, like the economic life, on opportunistic relationships based on geography. The form of these relationships will only develop in a healthy way when the national is born from freedom and not freedom born from the national. If one strives for freedom instead of nationalism then such striving is based on world-historical evolution. If one strives for nationalism then one is working against such evolution and plants the seed for new conflicts and wars. To demand of the leading statesmen of Austria that they should have abstained from delivering the ultimatum to Serbia means to demand of them that they should have acted against the interest of the country led by them. Theoreticians of all colours can make such demands. A person who reckons with existing facts should not seriously speak of such demands. If the southern Slavs had achieved what was wanted by leading greater Serbians, then, under the actions of the remaining Austrian Slavs, Austria would not have remained in the form in which it stood. In that case, one could imagine that Austria would have taken another form. But could one demand of a leading Austrian statesman that he wait in resignation for such an outcome? One could obviously only demand it if one were of the opinion that it belonged to the unconditional requirements of an Austrian statesman to be an absolute pacifist and to wait fatalistically for the fate of the empire. Under any other circumstances one must understand the step of Austria respecting the ultimatum.

3. Once Austria had given the ultimatum, the further sequence of events was only stoppable if Russia remained passive. As soon as Russia took an aggressive step the further sequence of events was unstoppable.

4. It is equally true that everyone who reckoned with the facts in Germany had the feeling that if once the indicated entanglements moved to a critical phase then there would be war. One could not escape this. And persons in position of responsibility were of the opinion that one must, if the war became necessary, conduct this war with full force. Certainly no one in Germany who really

came into consideration had the intention to start a war on their own initiative. One can demonstrate to the Entente that it did not have the slightest reason to believe in a war of aggression from the side of Germany. One can force them to acknowledge that they had the belief that Germany would become so powerful without war that this power would become dangerous to the current united powers of the Entente. One will, however, have to present such political evidence quite differently from how this has happened up to now, because this has not been political evidence but merely a list of political assertions which the others could choose to see as a show of brute force. It was believed from the side of the Entente powers that if the situation continued then one could not know what would yet become of Germany; therefore war with Germany would have to come. Germany could take the standpoint: we do not need war, but we will achieve without war that which the states of the Entente will not let us have without war; therefore we must be prepared for this war and when it threatens we will meet the situation so that we cannot be damaged by it. This is also valid in relation to the Serbian question and the Austrian question. Austria could no longer deal with Serbia in 1914 without a war — at least this must have been the conviction of its statesman. If the Entente had determined to let Austria-Hungary deal with Serbia, then it would not have had to come to the general war. Thus the true cause of the war ought not to be sought with the Central European powers, but rather in the fact that the Entente did not want to leave these Central

European powers in the power relationships as they existed in 1914. If, to be sure, the above-mentioned 'other action' had taken place before 1914, the Serbs would not have developed international opposition against Austria-Hungary and the ultimatum as well as the interference of Russia could not have happened. Had Russia turned against Central Europe purely for reasons of conquest at any other time, then it would have been impossible for England to act at its side. Since the submarine was a pure tool of war up to the war, but without this tool it would have been impossible for America to enter the war against the Central European powers, only England need be taken into account in the suggested sense as regards the peace question.

5. What should be communicated to the world now is:

a) Germany was completely taken by surprise by the events of July 1914 as far as the relevant personalities who had to decide about the outbreak of war were concerned — no one anticipated them. This holds true particularly of Russia's attitude.

b) In Germany any responsible reflection had to assume that if Russia attacked then France would also attack.

c) Germany had prepared its two-front war for many years with this situation in mind. If it did not receive a certain guarantee from the western powers that France would not attack Germany, then it could do nothing else in the process of these events that pressed in on one another than to initiate this two-front war. This guarantee could come only from England.

d) If England had given this guarantee, Germany would only have engaged in war against Russia.

e) German diplomacy believed as a result of the relations established with England in recent years that England would act to provide such a guarantee.

f) German diplomacy completely deceived itself with regard to the impending policy of England and under the impression of this deception the march through Belgium was initiated; if England had given the guarantees referred to, then Germany would have abstained from that action. In a completely unambiguous way the world should be told that the invasion of Belgium was only initiated when German diplomacy had been surprised by the communication from the English King that it would deceive itself if it waited for such a guarantee from England. It is incomprehensible why the German government does not do what it unambiguously could do, namely, to prove that the government would not have undertaken the invasion of Belgium if the decisive telegram from the King of England had read differently. The complete further course of the war truly depended on this decisive turn of events and Germany did not do anything in order to bring these decisive facts to the general attention of the world. If these facts had rightly been understood, one would indeed have to say that England's policy was falsely interpreted in Germany at decisive points, but one could not fail to recognize that England was the decisive factor in the Belgian question. If Germany presented these decisive facts to the world, a difficulty would arise with respect to Russia because Russia would perceive the debt it owed England for this war. This difficulty could only be removed if one were to succeed in demonstrating to Russia that it has less to expect from friendship with England than from friendship with Germany. This naturally cannot happen without Germany undertaking at the present time to develop a generous policy in association with Austria-Hungary through which Wilson's programme — presented to the world without knowledge of European circumstances — would be driven from the field.

It may appear practical to say there is no value today in speaking about the origins of the war. But it is the most impractical thing that can be imagined in the face of the actual situation. Because actually the Entente has waged the war for a long time with its description of its origins. It owes the situation which it has created to the circumstance that its characterization is believed. Fundamentally it is believed for the reason that Germany has not developed an effective response. While Germany could show that it has contributed nothing to the outbreak of the war, that it was driven into violating Belgian neutrality only through the conduct of England, the official position of Germany has been framed such that no person living outside Germany is prevented from forming the judgement that it rested in Germany's hands not to begin the war. Assembling the documents as was done is not sufficient. Such a collection of documents results in something that can be doubted by anyone while an unvarnished presentation of the facts would show Germany's innocence. People who have an understanding of such things know that the German description as given by people in positions of responsibility in Germany is not comprehended by the psyche of the people in the enemy and neutral countries and therefore is only taken as concealing the truth. One would only have the right to say that there is no point in speaking differently in the face of the hate of the enemy if one had made the attempt really to speak differently. One should not even think about using this hate as an excuse because that would be naïve. This hate is only the drapery of the war; it is only the slimy creation of those who want or have to accompany the unspeakably sad events of this war with their speeches or of those who seek through incitement of such hate an effective means of achieving this or that end. France and Russia are waging this war for reasons which are sufficiently well known. England is simply waging a war of economics — but an economic war which is a result of all that which has been prepared in England for a long time. To speak of the policy of isolation of King Edward and similar trivialities in the face of the reality of English politics is like seeing a young boy running away from a wooden stake. Afterwards the stake falls over and the young boy is accused of making the wooden stake fall over because he shook it a little bit. In fact the wooden stake had long since been so damaged that it only needed a slight collision from the boy finally to make it fall. The truth is that England managed for many years to pursue a policy guided by real knowledge of the

situation in Europe. England followed this policy in a way
it saw as favourable to itself out of a kind of natural
scientific exploitation of the forces available in the states
and peoples. Nowhere except in England did politics
carry such a wholly pertinent and self-coherent character.
Take the driving forces of the Balkan peoples, combine
them with events in Austria and then observe from the
perspective of these facts the political formulas that
existed in initiated circles in England. These formulas
always stated: this and that will happen in the Balkans
and England will respond with certain actions. The events
moved in the indicated direction and English policy
moved in parallel with them. One could find in England
sayings incorporated in such formulas as: the Russian
Empire in its current form will perish in order that the
Russian people will be able to live. These peoples are so
formed in their circumstances that one will be able to
conduct socialist experiments there for which there is no
chance in Western Europe. Anyone who follows English
policy can see that it was always prepared on a large scale
to turn these and many other events to the benefit of
England, profiting from the fact that it alone in all of
Europe proceeded from such a position and thus creating
its diplomatic advantage. England's policies were constantly put at the service of the real forces of the state and
its people, and its striving was to make these forces serve
itself to its economic advantage. It worked to its own
advantage. Of course others do that also. In addition to
working out of real knowledge of the forces of other

peoples and states, England worked out of real knowledge of the forces that lie in England. Other countries did not engage in the observation of such forces. Indeed, people in the other countries would only have smiled politely if one had talked to them about such forces. England's whole state structure is adapted to such real practical work. Others will only be able to unfold statesmanship equal to England's when that which has been indicated is no longer an English secret but common property. Just imagine how endlessly naïve it was when people believed that they could prevail from Germany with the Baghdad railway issue. From Germany they tackled the problem as if it just would be necessary to set about the work as one begins with the construction of a domestic road; one just comes to an understanding with one's neighbours about the project. Or to speak of something farther afield, how did Austria imagine it would put in order its Balkan relationships without marshalling forces that, conceived from the perspective of the state and national forces of the Balkans, could paralyse England's trumps? At any given moment England did not just do this and that; it controlled the international forces such that they went in England's favour at the right time. To accomplish this, one must first be acquainted with these forces and then develop oneself what is appropriate to these forces. Austria-Hungary would have had to accomplish an act at the right moment that would have turned the southern Slav forces in Austria's direction in a manner consistent with the nature of these forces. Germany would have had to turn the Baghdad railway interests in its direction in a manner consistent with the economic and opportunistic forces. Instead the southern Slav forces were deflected in the Russian direction and thereby in the Russian-English direction. The Baghdad railway was deflected in the English direction.

The war in Central Europe must lead to people becoming insightful to what exists in the national, state and economic life. By this alone can England be compelled no longer to conduct itself by way of superior diplomacy towards other states but instead to negotiate as an equal among equals about that which is to be negotiated among communities in Europe. Without fulfilling this condition, all imitation of the English parliament in Central Europe is nothing other than a means of throwing sand in one's own eyes. Otherwise, in England a number of persons will always find ways and means to let their reality-based policies be implemented through their parliament. Having a matter decided by an assembly of 500 instead of by a few statesmen is not enough in itself to make German and Austrian behaviour clever. One can hardly imagine anything more unfortunate than the superstition that it would work miracles if use of the English democratic model were added to everything else one has put up with from England. This should not be taken to mean that Central Europe should not undergo inner political development. Only such a development should not be the imitation of the Western European so-called democracy. Instead this development must precisely bring that which such

democracy would hinder in Central Europe because of
Central Europe's particular situation. This so-called
democracy is only suited to making the people of Central
Europe part of Anglo-American hegemony. If one also
had dealings with the so-called inter-country organizations of the present internationalists, then one would have
the nice prospect of being constantly overruled as a Central European in this inter-country organization.

What matters is to show the impulses that arise from
Central European life and that are truly of Central Europe.
When these impulses are revealed and seen by the western antagonists, they will see that they must bleed to
death on them if they further prosecute the war. These
antagonists can set their power against pretensions of
power on the part of the Germans and will so do, so long
as the Germans retain these pretensions. Faced with true
power the antagonists will surrender their weapons.
Wilson's effective manifesto must be opposed by what in
Central Europe can really be done for the liberation of the
life of the people because Wilson's words are not capable
of giving the people anything but Anglo-American hegemony. It is not necessary for Central Europe to seek harmony with Russia by a programme based on reality,
because this harmony will result automatically. Such a
Central European programme must not contain anything
that is only related to internal affairs of state but must
concentrate on external relations. But of course these
things must be seen in a suitable manner, because whether
a person can think well is certainly a matter of his inner

organization — but whether through this good thinking he works outward in this or that direction is not an inner matter.

Therefore only a Central European programme which is real can defeat Wilson's programme. That means a programme that does not stress some wishful idea but rather is simply a transcription of that which Central Europe can do because it has the power to do it in itself. This includes:

1. An understanding that the object of a democratic representation of the people can only be purely political, military and police matters. These are only possible on the basis of the historically developed substratum. If these issues are represented in a people's representative body and managed by a civil service responsible to this body, then these issues will necessarily develop conservatively. An external proof is that since the outbreak of the war even the Social Democrats have become conservative in these matters. And the Social Democrats will become yet more conservative the more they are forced to conceive in the appropriate terms that only ˙political, military and police concerns can be the object of such a people's representative body. Within such an arrangement the German individuality can also develop its system as a federal state which is not an incidental matter but something that is part of the character of the German people.

2. All economic issues are organized in a specific economic parliament. When the latter is relieved of all political and military concerns, then it will handle its affairs

purely in the way that is solely appropriate to them, namely, opportunistically. The civil service administration for these economic issues, within whose domain also lies the full administration of tariff laws, is directly responsible only to the economic parliament.

3. All juridical, pedagogical and spiritual concerns are in the free hands of the individual. In this domain the state only has the right to police, not the right to initiate. What is meant here only appears to be radical. In reality only someone who cannot look with unprejudiced eyes will be offended by the intention here. The state leaves it to the business, professional and ethnic organizations to establish their courts of justice, their schools, their churches and so forth and it leaves it to the individual to determine for himself his school, his church, his judge (naturally not from case to case but over a period of time). In the beginning such a development will have to be limited by territorial boundaries. Yet it contains the possibility of settling national and global antagonisms by peaceful means. It even carries the possibility of creating something real in place of the shadowy court of arbitration of nations. National or other agitators would be completely deprived of influence. No Italian in Trieste would find supporters in this city if everyone could develop their national forces there, notwithstanding that for evident opportunistic reasons their economic interests are arranged in Vienna and their policemen are paid from there.

The political structures of Europe could develop on the

basis of a sound conservatism that would never be intent on a partition of Austria but at most on its expansion.

The economic structures would develop in a sound opportunistic fashion because nobody would want to have Trieste in an economic structure in which it had to fail, since nobody would be hindered by the economy from participating in his religion, national group and so on according to his own choice.

Cultural affairs would be freed from the pressure that comes from the economic and political domains and cultural affairs would stop bringing pressure to bear on politics and the economy. All these cultural affairs are continuously maintained in healthy change.

A kind of senate—elected from the three bodies that have the task of ordering the political-military, the economic, the judicial-educational affairs—looks after the common interests, including, for example, the joint finances.

The feasibility of what is described here will not be doubted by anyone who thinks on the basis of the real situation in Central Europe. For nothing is called for here that must be implemented; the sole intention is to illustrate what is waiting for implementation and what will succeed in the very moment that the green light is given.

If one understands this, then it becomes clear why we have this war and why the war under the false flag of national liberation is really a war for the oppression of the German people and, in a wider sense, a war for the

oppression of all independent national life in Central
Europe. If one lays bare Wilson's programme, the latest
manifestation of the embracing programmes of the
Entente, then one discovers that its implementation would
mean nothing but the destruction of Central European
freedom. This is true in spite of Wilson speaking about the
freedom of the people because the world does not conform to words but to facts that follow from the realization
of these words. Central Europe needs true freedom but
Wilson does not speak of true freedom at all. The entire
Western world has absolutely no idea of the true freedom
that is necessary for Central Europe. It speaks of freedom
of the people and means by that not the true freedom of
individuals but rather a chimera like collective freedom of
groups of people as they have developed in Western
European states and in America. In the special circumstances of Central Europe such collective freedom cannot
be the result of the international situation and thus such
collective freedom must never at any time be the subject of
international agreements as, for instance, the conclusion of
peace can be subject of such agreements. In Central Europe the collective freedom of peoples must result from
general human freedom, and the latter will result if one
opens the way for general human freedom by detaching
everything that does not belong to the purely political,
military and economic life. It is no great surprise that those
who always reckon only with their ideas and not with
realities will raise the kind of objections against such a
separation as can be found in a recently published book,

Krieck's *Die deutsche Staatsidee*. On page 167 it says:
'Occasionally in the past the demand was made by,
among others, E. von Hartmann to create an economic
parliament alongside the people's assembly. This idea is
completely in line with economic and social developments. But apart from the fact that a new, big cog would
increase the already substantial clumsiness and friction of
the machine, the responsibilities of the two parliaments
would be impossible to demarcate.'

However, as far as this idea is concerned, it should be
admitted that it arises on the real basis of developments
and that it must therefore be implemented. It should not
be rejected in a move counter to developments because its
realization might be found difficult. If one stops making
progress in real developments in the face of such difficulties, then one creates entanglements that later discharge violently. And, after all, this war represents in its
specific manifestation the discharge of difficulties that
were not resolved in the right ways while there was still
time to do so.

The Wilson programme aims to make impossible in
the world the legitimate tasks and existential conditions
of the Central European states. The Wilson programme
must be contrasted with what will happen in Central
Europe if such events are not interrupted by a violent
destruction of Central European existence. Wilson's programme must be confronted with what only Central
Europe can do on the basis of what has evolved here
historically if it does not unite with the Entente, which

cannot have any interest in guiding Central Europe towards its natural development.

As things are today, Austria and Germany only have a choice among the following three:

1. To wait under all circumstances for a military victory and to hope that this will bring the possibility of carrying out their Central European tasks.

2. To enter a peace with the Entente on the basis of the present programme and thereby to face certain destruction.

3. To say in the light of the true circumstances what they view as the result of peace, thereby giving the world the opportunity of letting nations choose, through clear understanding of the circumstances and the intentions of Central Europe, between, on the one hand, a fact-based programme of peace that brings the people of Europe true freedom and thus of course freedom to nations, or, on the other hand, an illusory programme from the West and America which speaks of freedom but in reality makes existence impossible for all Europe. We in Central Europe give the impression at the moment that we shrink from saying to the West what we should want while the West shows no reluctance to overwhelm us with the manifestation of its will. Thus the West gives the impression of being the only one to want to heal humankind while we have striven solely to destroy the West's praiseworthy endeavours by militarism and other means. Yet it is the West—having through this impression prepared a long

while, and continuing to prepare still better, to give us a shadow existence — which is in truth the creator of our militarism. Certainly such and similar things have often been said. But we arrive at nothing from such things being said by some person or other. We will only achieve something when these ideas become the leitmotiv of European actions and when the world learns to recognize that they can expect no other kind of action from Central Europe except such that must draw the sword when someone forces the sword into its hand. The development of German militarism, as it is called by the nations of the West, has been forged by the latter over hundreds of years and only they and not Germany can be responsible for creating a situation in which it is no longer needed. However, it is the responsibility of Central Europe clearly to present its will for freedom, a will that is not built in a Wilson fashion on programmes but on the reality of the human existence.

There is therefore only one peace programme for Central Europe: to let the world know that peace is possible immediately if the Entente replaces its current dishonest peace programme with one that is honest in that it provides for Central Europe to exist rather than its downfall. All other questions that may become the subject of a peace endeavour resolve themselves when they are approached on the basis of these assumptions. The basis that is offered to us by the Entente and which has been taken up by Wilson makes peace impossible. If no alternative is found, then the German people can only be brought by force to acceptance of this programme and the further course of European history will demonstrate the correctness of what has been said because the realization of Wilson's programme will bring the European peoples to ruin. One must view the situation in Central Europe without illusion with regard to what those personalities have believed for so many years and considered from their point of view as the law of world development: that the Anglo-American race owns the future of world development and that it should take over responsibility for the inheritance of the Latin race and for the education of the Russian race. When an Englishman or American who deems himself to be initiated sets out this geo-political formula, it is always made clear that the German element should have no say in the ordering of the world because of its insignificance in world political matters, that the Latin element does not need to be considered because it will die out in any case, and that the Russian element has someone who makes himself into this element's educator. One would not need to think too much of such a confession of faith if it lived in the heads of a few people inclined to political fantasy or Utopia. Yet English politics uses countless means to make this programme into the practical content of its real global policy, and from the perspective of England the present coalition—in which it finds itself—could not be better suited for turning this programme into reality. There is nothing with which Central Europe can oppose it other than a programme of true human liberation that could be realized at any time if human beings would find the will to do so. One might perhaps think that peace will take a long time to arrive, even if the programme referred to here is put before the European people, since it will not be possible to put it into practice during the war. Moreover, the Entente would maintain that the programme had been presented by Central European leaders to the nations to deceive them and that therefore after the war the terrible things would simply recur which they would have to 'remove once and for all in the struggle for the freedom and rights of nations' on moral grounds. But anyone who judges the world correctly according to facts and not according to his favourite opinions must know that everything that accords with reality has a very different persuasive power from what arises out of pure arbitrariness. And one can quietly await what will be revealed among those people who can see for themselves that with the Central European programme the Entente nations only lose the possibility of crushing Central Europe, but nothing flows from it that is irreconcilable with the true existential impulse of the nations of the Entente. So long as one remains in the region of masked intentions, understanding will be impossible; as soon as one shows the realities behind the mask, not only the military but also the political realities, a very different form of events will begin. The world has become acquainted with the weapons of Central Europe for Central Europe's well-being. Central Europe's political intentions remain a book with seven seals to the world. Instead the world receives a daily image of how horrible and worthy of destruction

Central Europe is. And it appears to the world as if Central Europe remains silent before this frightening image, which must of course appear to the world as an acknowledgment of the same.

Of course countless issues arise for anyone who really thinks about how the programme indicated here should be put into practice in detail. Yet these issues only arise if the programme is thought of as something to be realized by an individual or a society. But it would refute itself if it were conceived in this way. It should be thought of as the expression of what the peoples of Central Europe will do if the governments set themselves the task to recognize and free the forces of the people. What will happen in detail always shows itself in such things when they are on the way to being realized. Then they are not precepts for something that has to happen but rather predictions of what will happen if one lets things proceed along the path demanded by their own nature. And with regard to all religious and spiritual cultural relationships, to which national culture also belongs, this individual nature dictates administration by cultural organizations to which the individual person commits himself out of free will and which will be administered in the parliament of cultural organizations as a cultural organization such that the parliament concerns itself with the cultural organizations themselves but never with the relation between this cultural organization and the individual person. And never should an organization deal with a person belonging to another organization in the same field. Such a cultural organization would be accepted into the parliament of cultural organizations when it united a specific number of people. Until then it would remain a private affair in which no administrative or representative body could interfere. Whoever finds it distasteful that from this perspective cultural-spiritual affairs would in future no longer be subject to special privileges must put up with it for the benefit of society. From the ever-growing habituation to special privileges, people in many circles will find it difficult to accept the need to leave behind special privileges, especially for professions like education, medicine, law and religion, and return to the venerated ancient idea of the free spiritual-cultural organization. The cultural organizations should see to it that a person becomes qualified for his profession but also that the practice of these professions should not be a matter of special privileges but rather should come about by free competition and free human choice. That will be difficult to accept, particularly for those who like to say that people are not mature enough to deal with any given issue. In reality this objection will not have to be considered in any case, because, with the exception of the necessarily free professions, the cultural organization will decide on the applicants. Equally, no difficulties can arise in the relationship with the political and economic spheres that could not be solved in reality in the implementation of the intended objectives. How educational institutions are set up, for example, which in their regulations touch on the two representative bodies not concerned with education as such, would be a matter for the superior-level senate.

Second Memorandum of 1917 — Final Version

'No people must be forced under a sovereignty under which it does not wish to live. No territory must change hands except for the purpose of securing those who inhabit it a fair chance of life and liberty ... And then the free peoples of the world must draw together in common covenant ... that will in effect combine their forces to secure peace and justice in the dealings of nations with one another. The brotherhood of mankind must no longer be a fair but empty phrase: it must be given a structure of force and reality.'[45] So Mr W. Wilson describes what through the American participation in this war is to become reality. These are attractive words, about which one can say that every reasonable person with healthy common sense must acknowledge them. If these words had been composed by a literary idealist to please a circle of readers, one could simply acknowledge them as a matter of course. One could state with the attitude of the moralist that whoever objects to these words cannot be a friend of progress and freedom. One can already today hear voices that stress that the war has brought this lesson: only those who acknowledge such or similar ideas and direct their actions towards them now practise higher, contemporary politics.

Speaking about 'opinions' and about how this or that opinion must be advocated because of a person's belief will never lead to a basis for practical action. It is only of use to look clearly at practical deeds. For the inhabitants of the Central European states no discussion about the 'general human' justification of the Entente's goals, that is to say about the 'beauty' of these goals, can be of any worth, but only an understanding of the true power relationship established by these goals in the life of nations. Therefore in what follows we will look at the true form of the Entente's aims for Europe without consideration of whether what will be said sounds pleasant to the leaders of the Entente. Only through such an orientation of thinking can one arrive at practical impulses. The things will be somewhat sharply formulated because they must be for the reason stated. It should be explicitly noted that the present moods will play no role in this formulation, but rather alone the clear-headed observation of the facts of the last decade. Understanding what the Entente intends must be the foundation for the principles found in Central Europe; to be blinded by what it says leads to the worst of false paths.

It is in any case an unthankful task to be forced to have to turn against ideas that seem to have won the hearts and minds of people to a high degree; which, moreover, seem to be the result of 'the true historical development of humanity toward noble democracy'. Yet what follows must be built on the foundation that the acknowledgment of Wilson's intentions must not only make a mockery of logic for those who belong to the Central and Eastern European peoples, but also that during and after the war every single activity and measure must happen in such a way that these intentions of Wilson and the Entente must break themselves on the health and fruitfulness of these measures and activities.

The Entente's real war aims have been veiled in a questionable way in the manner in which Mr Wilson gives expression to his intentions. One cannot avoid dealing with the former when dealing with the latter. Achieving the cleverest conceptual refutation of the Wilson 'programme' is not of relevance at this time. We are not currently dealing with arguments to distinguish who is right and who is not. In the area with which we are here concerned the only thing of value is what happens or has the potential to make things happen. And thoughts that are thought and spoken of as seeds for present and future actions only have value when they are carried in the sense here indicated. Wilson's words are not spoken by a literary friend of humanity. They are the banner to which the Americans are arming themselves, and the deeds that the Entente have accomplished against Central Europe over the last three years. The facts are that Central Europe has to fight against that which is proclaimed under this banner as going into battle for the benefit of humanity, for the liberation of peoples. The Entente and Wilson say what they allege they are fighting for. These words have the power of advertisement. The power of their advertisement becomes progressively more serious. There are people in

Central Europe that surely will not admit that they are repeating Wilson's words, yet their ideas are not dissimilar to his words. Anyone who knows the origins of the war in a deeper sense cannot but stress the necessity that the Wilson-Entente programme in Central Europe should suffer the sharpest rejection through the facts. Because the real prospects of this programme — next to its causing moral blindness — lie in its wanting to use the instincts of Central and Eastern European peoples to manipulate them unconsciously by moral and political means towards economic dependence on the Anglo-Americans. Anyone who knows that in circles of English initiates the 'coming world war' was spoken about since the last century as the event that must bring the Anglo-American race to world dominance, cannot take seriously that leaders of the Entente claim they were surprised or wanted to prevent the war even if these assurances by the leaders, as they are expressed at the moment, may be subjectively true for them. Those who spoke of the 'coming world war' as an inevitable event count on the true historical forces of European peoples. They count on the instincts of the Europeans, namely, the Slavic people. And they wanted to guide and use the ideals of the Slavic peoples in such a way that they would become of service to the national egotism of the Anglo-Americans. They count further on the decline of the Latin world on whose ruins they want to build their own empire. They thus count on the large-scale historic perspectives of peoples and nations that they want to bring into the service of their own goals. And these goals lead to the purpose of crushing the Central European state structures, however strongly this is denied from the side of the Entente. It is right to emphasize in a completely clear-headed fashion that the goal of the leaders of the Entente is to crush Central Europe because the only possible response to the very effective statements of the Entente is to emphasize this goal. But a response which is negative because it wants to refute what is said by the Entente has no value. Therefore the following answer will be positive which means pointing to the facts that oppose the Entente from Central Europe.

Only by the recognition that this is so can Central Europe bring those impulses that will lead out of the chaos of the present. The Central European state grouping can only adopt the position of making the programme of the Entente unworkable by taking appropriate measures. This Entente programme — more or less spoken or unspoken — rests on three propositions:

1. that the historically developed European state grouping must not — from the standpoint of the Entente — be recognized as the ones which are responsible for solving the European ethnic problems;

2. that the Central European state grouping must not compete with the Anglo-Americans but should, rather, be in a relationship of dependence.

3. that the cultural-spiritual relations of Central and Eastern Europe will be ordered in the interest of Anglo-American national egotism.

Only someone who is able to recognize that the translation of these three points into the Wilson-Entente language is the same as used by Wilson in his letter to the Russians is able to see through what is happening.

It may also be that through the pressure of events we will get peace in the near future. Perhaps this will happen if England sees that it cannot any longer sustain itself at the moment without consenting to ending the war. All that does not alter the essentials on the Anglo-American side. If the Anglo-Americans find it possible to continue the war, then they will continue to clothe the three above points in the formula of Wilson's letter: 'For these are things we have always professed to desire, and unless we pour out the blood and treasure now and succeed, we may never be able to unite or show conquering force again in the great cause of human liberty.'[46] If the leading powers in England are obliged to allow the war to end in the near future then the future policies, which would remain oriented to the above three points, would be formulated: 'We wanted to sacrifice money and blood for human liberation, we have done it in a high degree while the Central European powers have been intent only on the opposite. We have for the time being only partially prevailed against these powers. Our goal stands undiminished before our eyes because it is the goal of mankind.'

The true content of these intentions will only be countered if in Central Europe practical action is taken according to this knowledge: in the West people call domination by the Anglo-Americans human liberation and democracy. And because this is done, the impression is created as if there was a true wish to liberate humanity.

To prevail against the effects of this appalling deception, against the effects of an innate racial egotism clothed in an impossible morality, Central Europe must concentrate its approach on the full truth of the matter. And this truth is:

1. With the achievement of the Entente goals regarding the Central European state grouping, true European freedom is lost. For this state grouping could realize freedom because freedom lies in its own interest and states cannot act otherwise than holding their own interests in view. Anglo-Americanism cannot realize this national freedom because as soon as it exists it opposes the interest of the Anglo-American state grouping as long as this interest remains as it now is. This interest has given the war its stamp out of factual necessity. The Anglo-American states must come to the insight that they must respect the interests of the Central European states next to their own, and they must leave to the Central European states the ordering of the freedom of Central European peoples who alone can see as their true state interest the furthering of this freedom.

2. From the Central European perspective this war is an ethnic war when looking to the East and an economic war when looking to the West, to England and America. The war of revenge against France has only become possible through mixing up the revenge idea with the Anglo-

American economic interest and the Russian-Slav national ideas.

3. The liberation of peoples is possible. But it can only be the result and not the basis of individual freedom. If individuals are free, then nations will be free through them. If Central Europe wants to, it can act according to these three fundamental principles. And its action will become a programme of facts; it will act in this way if it implements an objective programme for individual freedom in contrast to the Entente-Wilson programme, which without any knowledge at all of the forces of the Central European people speaks of something that is not existent in the world of facts but only in the aspirations of Anglo-American racial egotism. The programme here considered the right programme for Central Europe is not radical in the sense that people in many circles shrink back from radicalism. It is, rather, only an expression of facts wanting to realize themselves through their own force in Central Europe. They should be realized with full consciousness and not be kept concealed in order to be realized through their own nature in the fog of the Entente-Wilson goals, where they would become corrupted and thereby become the incentive and excuse for further warlike entanglements.

Their true realization will never happen if that which must be the intention of Central Europe remains concealed through the unnatural mixing of political, economic and general human interests.

The political circumstances demand healthy conservatism in the sense of preservation and consolidation of the historically developed state systems if these circumstances are to flourish. The economic and general human interests bristle against this conservatism, which is a vital necessity for Central Europe, only so long as they have to suffer through being mixed with the conservative state systems. And the political conservatism, when it thinks of its true interests, does not have the slightest cause to continuously let itself be disturbed by being thrown together with the economic and general human interests. If this mixing is stopped, then the economic and general human interests will reconcile themselves with the political conservatism and the latter can quietly develop according to its own being.

Economic relations require opportunism, which manages the organization of economic relations according to its own nature, in order to flourish. It must lead to conflict if economic measures stand in a relationship to political and general human requirements that is different from their own appropriate laws and administration in their natural context. Here we do not mean only conflict within the state, but mainly conflict that discharges externally in political difficulties and explosions of war.

General human relations and the related question of national freedom must be built on individual freedom now and in the future. In this matter one will not be able to make a beginning with relevant observations as long as one believes that freedom or liberation of peoples could be spoken about without it being built upon the freedom of the individual, and as long as one does not understand that with the true freedom of the individual the freedom of the peoples is necessarily provided because it happens as the natural result of the former. The individual must be able to commit himself to a people, to a religious community, to any association that arises from his general human aspirations without being held back in his commitment by his political or economic associations through state structures.

What matters is to understand that all forms of historically developed state structures are able to accomplish the liberation of human beings when they are directed to it through their own interest, which is exactly the case with the Central European states. A parliamentary development of these states may be seen as necessary for reasons of contemporary developments and of popular feeling. Only the threefold state structure as described can address the question that must be thrown into the world's public arena now because of the confusion of war. Merely asking for parliamentarianism changes nothing in the circumstances that have led to the present chaos. The western nations speak so much about parliamentarianism because they understand nothing of Central European circumstances. They give themselves over to the belief that what is considered to be right for their interests must serve as a pattern for the entire world. What is valid for Central Europe, even if parliamentarianism should rule, is a parliamentarianism in which the political, the economic and the general human relations can unfold independently of one another in legislation and administration, and thereby support one another instead of entangling themselves in their outward effects and creating conflicts. Central Europe frees itself and the world from such conflicts when it excludes such mutual interference of the three human realms in life from its state structures. The goals of the Entente and Wilson can be no match for the power that will be exhibited by Central Europe if it presents to the world that of which only it is capable and which no one else can bring forth. Human and thus national liberation would be presented to the world as a necessary part of the instinct of the Central European states and peoples if they, as here indicated, are thrown into the events of the present as authentic and factual impulses.

What is here described should not be imagined as a Utopian programme; it is not intended to eliminate historical rights and legal structures. To anyone who examines it closely, it represents something that with full awareness of all historical rights and by recognition of factual circumstances can grow without any concerns out of the present state structures. It is self-evident that what has been presented here cannot consider the details. Such details reveal themselves in true practical impulses only in the execution. Only a Utopian could invent the details, and therefore his assertions, which arise from abstract thinking, could not be realized. What is here said should only appear in general outline. But these outlines are not thought out but rather observed from Central European circumstances. That guarantees that they will hold true exactly when they are to be applied in practice as outlined. What is here discussed is in a certain sense already a necessity of life. The question is only how to serve this necessity. Neither is it necessary to speak about the details now because it is an internal affair of the Central European states. At present it is only necessary to present as much of the issue to the world as has meaning externally. What matters is to show the impulses that truly lie in Central European life, and to so show it in such a way that the Western antagonists see that they will find themselves opposing indestructible impulses if they continue to prosecute the war. Thereby something will be set in opposition to the leaders of the Entente, not simply proposed, which to date has not been set against them, and which they cannot master through any war programme from their side. A language, as is here meant, that carries the seeds of reality in itself, when spoken before the world must have consequences. The settlement with Russia does not need to be considered now in connection with our current deliberations because such a settlement will result by itself in due course as a consequence. And the understanding that such a result will occur will ripen impulses in the Russian leadership that only can have favourable results. It must always be taken into consideration that what is here indicated is not at first of importance as an internal affair of the state. Rather, what is important is its outward manifestation in the present world conflict with regard to the conclusion of the conflict, namely, in a political struggle with the manifestations of the leadership of the Entente and Wilson. The internal aspect, in this case, comes to consideration in a similar way as the deeds that arise from a person's thinking are realities for other people, despite the fact that how a person thinks is only an inner matter for him. It is only necessary for a person to explain the results of his thinking to others and not his inner constitution.

Recognizing and accepting the division of political, economic and general human domains in legislation, administration and social structures as the goal of Central European striving will paralyse the forces of the West. That will force the western powers to think themselves into a situation alongside the European central powers, and the eastern powers that cooperate with them under these circumstances, in which the western powers confine themselves within the limits of their national instincts to giving only themselves state structures that suit themselves. The central and eastern peoples are allowed to live their shared community in the sense of true individual freedom within their natural regions without the kind of interference which existed as the cause of the war — while at the moment the western powers believe they can present their own purposes as the decisive factor in the world conflict.

It all depends on understanding how differently the relations between states and peoples, and also individuals, will occur when these relations are based on the specific external effect that follows from the division of the three life factors, than if the conflicts which result from their confusion are entangled in these external effects. In the future, the history of the events leading up to this war will be written so that it will directly be shown how the war arose through the unfortunate reciprocal interference of these three areas of life in the intercourse between nations. By their separation, the forces of one area of life work outwardly to have a harmonizing effect on the others; the forces of economic interests especially balance out conflicts that arise on political grounds and the general human area of interest can unfold its community building forces, while the latter forces precisely will be driven to complete outer ineffectiveness if they have to make their appearance burdened with political and economic conflicts. Lately nothing has given rise to greater self-delusion than this last point. People did not see that general human relations can unfold their true force outwardly only if they are inwardly built upon the foundation of the free organization. They then work together with the economic interests in such a way that in the course of these effects something develops in a natural, living way which others want to give a dubious future through the creation of the Utopian structures of a super-state: Utopian courts of arbitration, a Wilsonian 'League of Nations' and so forth, that can lead to nothing but continuous out-voting of Central Europe by the other states. Such things suffer from the mistake under which everything suffers when wished abstractions are forced upon the facts while, through the path here indicated, development is given a free road that is actually striven for out of the facts themselves and which therefore can be realized.

If one understands this, then it becomes clear why we have this war and why the war under the false flag of national liberation is really a war for the oppression of the German people and, in a wider sense, a war for the oppression of all independent national life in Central Europe. If one lays bare Wilson's programme, the latest manifestation of the embracing programmes of the Entente, then one discovers that its implementation would mean nothing but the destruction of Central European freedom. This is true in spite of Wilson speaking about the freedom of the people because the world does not conform to words but to facts that follow from the realization of these words. Central Europe needs true freedom but Wilson does not speak of true freedom at all. The entire western world has absolutely no idea of the true freedom that is necessary for Central Europe. It speaks of freedom of the people and means by that not the true freedom of individuals but rather a chimera like collective freedom of groups of people as they have developed in Western European states and in America. In the special circumstances of Central Europe such collective freedom cannot be the result of the international situation and thus such collective freedom must never at any time be the subject of international agreements as for instance the conclusion of peace can be the subject of such agreements. In Central Europe the collective freedom of peoples must result from general human freedom, and the latter will result if one opens the way for general human freedom by detaching everything that does not belong to the purely political, military and economic life. It is no great surprise that those who always reckon only with their ideas and not with realities will raise the kind of objections against such a separation as can be found in a recently published book, Krieck's *Die deutsche Staatsidee*. On page 167 it says: 'Occasionally in the past the demand was made by, among others, E. von Hartmann to create an economic parliament alongside the people's assembly. This idea is completely in line with economic and social developments. But apart from the fact that a new, big cog would increase the already substantial clumsiness and friction of the machine, the responsibilities of the two parliaments would be impossible to demarcate.'

However, as far as this idea is concerned, it should be admitted that it arises on the real basis of developments and that it must therefore be implemented. It should not be rejected in a move counter to developments because its realization might be found difficult. If one stops making progress in real developments in the face of such difficulties, then one creates entanglements that later discharge violently. And, after all, this war represents in its specific manifestation the discharge of difficulties that were not resolved in the right ways while there was still time to do so.

The Wilson programme aims to make impossible in the world the legitimate tasks and existential conditions of the Central European states. The Wilson programme must be contrasted with what will happen in Central Europe if such events are not interrupted by a violent destruction of Central European existence. Wilson's programme must be confronted with what only Central Europe can do on the basis of what has evolved here historically if it does not unite with the Entente, which cannot have any interest in guiding Central Europe towards its natural development.

As things are today, Austria and Germany only have a choice among the following three:

1. To wait under all circumstances for a military victory and to hope that this will bring the possibility of carrying out their Central European tasks.

2. To enter a peace with the Entente on the basis of the present programme and thereby to face certain destruction.

3. To say in the light of the true circumstances what they view as the result of peace, thereby giving the world the opportunity of letting nations choose, through clear understanding of the circumstances and the intentions of Central Europe, between, on the one hand, a fact-based programme of peace that brings the people of Europe true freedom and thus of course freedom to nations, or, on the other hand, an illusory programme from the West and America which speaks of freedom but in reality makes existence impossible for all Europe. We in Central Europe give the impression at the moment that we shrink from saying to the West what we should want while the West shows no reluctance to overwhelm us with the manifes-

tation of its will. Thus the West gives the impression of being the only one to want to heal humankind while we have striven solely to destroy the West's praiseworthy endeavours by militarism and other means. Yet it is the West—having through this impression prepared a long while, and continuing to prepare still better, to give us a shadow existence—which is in truth the creator of our militarism. Certainly such and similar things have often been said. But we arrive at nothing from such things being said by some person or other. We will only achieve something when these ideas become the leitmotiv of European actions and when the world learns to recognize that they can expect no other kind of action from Central Europe except such that must draw the sword when someone forces the sword into its hand. The development of German militarism, as it is called by the nations of the West, has been forged by the latter over hundreds of years and only they and not Germany can be responsible for creating a situation in which it is no longer needed. However, it is the responsibility of Central Europe clearly to present its will for freedom, a will that is not built in a Wilson fashion on programmes but on the reality of the human existence.

There is therefore only one peace programme for Central Europe: to let the world know that peace is possible immediately if the Entente replaces its current dishonest peace programme with one that is honest in that it provides for Central Europe to exist rather than its downfall. All other questions that may become the subject of a peace endeavour resolve themselves when they are approached on the basis of these assumptions. The basis that is offered to us by the Entente and which has been taken up by Wilson makes peace impossible. If no alternative is found, then the German people can only be brought by force to acceptance of this programme and the further course of European history will demonstrate the correctness of what has been said because the realization of Wilson's programme will bring the European peoples to ruin. One must view the situation in Central Europe without illusion with regard to what those personalities have believed for so many years and considered from their point of view as the law of world development: that the Anglo-American race owns the future of world development and that it should take over responsibility for the inheritance of the Latin race and for the education of the Russian race. When an Englishman or American who deems himself to be initiated sets out this geo-political formula, it is always made clear that the German element should have no say in the ordering of the world because of its insignificance in world political matters, that the Latin element does not need to be considered because it will die out in any case, and that the Russian element has someone who makes himself into this element's educator. One would not need to think too much of such a confession of faith if it lived in the heads of a few people inclined to political fantasy or Utopia. Yet English politics uses countless means to make this programme into the practical content of its real global policy, and from the perspective of England the present coalition—in which it finds itself—could not be better suited for turning this programme into reality. There is nothing with which Central Europe can oppose it other than a programme of true human liberation that could be realized at any time if human beings would find the will to do so. One might perhaps think that peace will take a long time to arrive, even if the programme referred to here is put before the European people, since it will not be possible to put it into practice during the war; moreover, the Entente would maintain that the programme had been presented by Central European leaders to the nations to deceive them and that therefore after the war the terrible things would simply recur which they would have to 'remove once and for all in the struggle for the freedom and rights of nations' on moral grounds. But anyone who judges the world correctly according to facts and not according to his favourite opinions must know that everything that accords with reality has a very different persuasive power from what arises out of pure arbitrariness. And one can quietly await what will be revealed among those people who can see for themselves that with the Central European programme the Entente nations only lose the possibility of crushing Central Europe, but nothing flows from it that is irreconcilable with the true existential impulse of the nations of the Entente. So long as one remains in the region of masked intentions, understanding will be impossible; as soon as one shows the realities behind the mask, not only the military but also the political realities, a very different form of events will begin. The world has become acquainted with the weapons of Central Europe for Central Europe's well-being. Central Europe's political intentions remain a book with seven seals to the world. Instead the world receives a daily image of how horrible and worthy of destruction Central Europe is. And it appears to the world as if Central Europe remains silent about this frightening image, which must of course appear to the world as an acknowledgment of the same.

It is understandable that there will be countless objections to what is presented here. These objections would only matter if what is here presented were viewed as a programme that should be accomplished by an individual or some society. But it is not intended in this way. It would refute itself if it were thought in this way. It is conceived as the expression of what the people of Central Europe will do if the governments set themselves the task of recognizing and liberating the forces of the people. What will happen in detail will always show itself in such things only when they are on the way to being realized. Then they are not precepts for something that has to happen but rather predictions of what will happen if one lets things proceed along the path demanded by their own nature. And with regard to all religious and spiritual cultural relationships to which also the national culture belongs, this own nature dictates administration through cultural organizations to which the individual person commits himself out of free will, and which will be administered in the parliament of cultural organizations as a cultural organization such that the parliament concerns itself with the cultural organizations concerned but never with the relation between this cultural organization and the individual person. Such a cultural organization would be accepted into the circle of the parliament of cultural organizations when it united a specific number of people. Until then it would remain a private affair in which no administrative or representative body could interfere. Whoever finds it distasteful that from this perspective cultural-spiritual affairs would in future no longer be subject to special privileges must put up with it for the benefit of society. From the ever-growing habituation to special privileges, people in many circles will find it difficult to accept the need to leave behind these special privileges, especially for professions like education, medicine, law and religion, and return to the venerated ancient idea of the free spiritual-cultural organization. The cultural organizations should see to it that a person becomes qualified for his profession but also that the practice of these professions should not be a matter of special privileges but rather should come about by free competition and free human choice. That will be difficult to accept, particularly for those who like to say that people are not mature enough to deal with any given issue. In reality this objection will not have to be considered in any case, because with the exception of the necessarily free professions the cultural organization will decide on the applicants. Equally, no difficulties can arise in the relationship with the political and economic spheres that could not be solved in reality in the implementation of the intended objectives. How educational institutions are set up, for example, which in their regulations touch on the two representative bodies not concerned with education as such, would be a matter for the superior-level senate.

All individual institutions as intended here can be achieved through the extension of historically given factors, which in no country of Central Europe need to be eliminated or radically replaced by other factors. The points can be found everywhere in what already exists which, when followed in the indicated direction, result in national liberation on the basis of individual freedom. To 'prove' that what is here stated is 'right' would be absurd because the rightness must arise from the fact of its realization. The next step would be the commitment to these impulses by persons in positions of authority. Nobody needs to be afraid that such an open declaration would in itself not already have an incredible positive effect for the European states. One can, on the contrary, quietly await what the leaders of the Entente will do (not say) when confronted with such an open commitment. With this commitment they must reckon differently than they have before with anything that comes from Central Europe. Until now they only needed to take Central European military successes into account; they should also be put in a position of having to take its political will into account.

Whoever thinks about what is suggested here in a truly practical sense, which means being in harmony with the actual circumstances, will be able to find that a foundation is created on which such complicated issues as the Austrian language question — including the official language and the lingua franca — and the German colonial question can rest. For what is proposed here will mitigate the error which so far has always been made, namely, that a resolution of such questions was considered before the factual foundation had been created on which such a resolution could be built. Until now people have tried to build the second floor without the first. This first floor for the Central European states is, however, the recognition of their lawful, necessary structure in conservative, historical, political representation and administration separated from the organization of the opportunistic economic element and the spiritual-cultural element. When one stands firmly on this ground, then one can begin to speak of parliamentarianism, democracy and similar things. These elements will not become different in themselves whether they are the expression of the unsustainable mix of political, economic and spiritual-cultural elements in Central Europe or the expression of their lawful structuring. Precisely through the effect that an open commitment held in this manner would bring about in the Entente leadership, one would see how, with such a commitment, one stands on the basis of real facts.

*

The practicability of what is presented here will not be doubted by anyone whose thinking is based in the true situation of Central Europe. For no programmes are being

demanded here but those things are being explained
which want to come to realization and which will succeed
in the moment that they are allowed to do so. If in place of
the Entente-Wilson peace formula its essence were to be
unmasked, then the following would come to light: 'We
Anglo-Americans want the world to become what we
wish it to be. Central Europe has to submit to this wish.'
This peace formula unmasked shows that Central Europe
was driven to war. If the Entente were to win it would
extinguish Central Europe's development. If Central
Europe adds the invincible weapon to its arsenal of the
peace offer to the world that it unconditionally intends to
realize what only Central Europe can realize—national
liberation through the liberation of the individual—then
Central Europe can set against the talk of 'the rights and
freedoms of nations' the factually true words: 'We fight
for our rights and our freedom and the realization of
human values that we can and will not let go. By its
nature, this realization impairs no true rights and freedoms of others. For what we want to become will carry a
guarantee of itself. If you nations of the West could come
to an understanding with us on these grounds and if you
nations of the East could comprehend that we do not want
anything different from you, if you first truly understand
yourselves, then freedom is possible tomorrow.'

5. The Metamorphosis of Intelligence

'The Metamorphosis of Intelligence' is a lecture of 15 December 1919 published in English for the first time in this volume.[47] It is different from the other texts in this volume in that the audience consisted of members of the Anthroposophical Society. Consequently, Steiner assumes a familiarity with his basic works, vocabulary and world-view. A sketch of the pertinent background is briefly provided in the footnotes to the text. It can also be gained by reading Steiner's Occult Science, An Outline *(Rudolf Steiner Press). The reason for including this text is that it gives an excellent sketch of the basics of Steiner's approach to a science of nations and nationalities. It contains some of his insights into what the different nationalities need to understand to work together harmoniously.*

In part of yesterday's lecture I took my start from an essay by Berdyaev, an essay based on the prejudice which we might describe as an unqualified belief in modern science and learning. This essay, however, also records a remarkable fact, intelligible only through the contrast between the logic of the intellect (which is of course the logic of modern science) and the logic of realities. Berdyaev points out that Bolshevism has appointed Avenarius, Mach and other noted positivists as its official philosophers so to speak. I may add explicitly that this essay was written as long ago as 1908. It is a remarkable thing—intelligible only on our spiritual-scientific basis—to find in the work of this Russian author a judgement (no matter what our attitude to these things may be) most in agreement with the present time, or perhaps I should rather say, a judgement still applicable to the present time. And it may be worth while for you to know that Mach and Avenarius were already referred to as official philosophers of the Bolsheviks at a time when—I hope I am making no undue assumptions—a considerable number possibly even of this audience had not the remotest idea what Bolshevism was. For a large part of humankind in Eastern and Central Europe have only been aware of the existence of Bolshevism for a very short time, whereas in fact it is a very old phenomenon.

I now want to add something more to the studies we have recently pursued. I was anxious above all to show you how the social impulses of the present time are to be judged and considered in the light of spiritual science. One thing we emphasized especially: we must not give ourselves up to the simple belief that the social impulses are to be conceived in a uniform way over the whole world. It will cloud and mislead all our thoughts and judgements about the social question if we do not take into account that human communities throughout the civilized world are differentiated. We must avoid the error into which we fall when we say of the social question that this or that holds good; human society must be ordered thus and thus. Rather, we must frame the question as follows: what is the nature of the forces in eastern humanity, what is the nature of the forces in western humanity, and what is their nature in the humanity living in the middle between the two? What is the nature in each case of the forces leading to the social demands of the age? We have already characterized in manifold ways, both from the external symptoms and from the inner esoteric standpoint, the nature of this differentiation between western humanity, central humanity, and eastern humanity; and observe that in the latter we include the European east, namely, Russia. We have already characterized how these differentiations are to be conceived. Without a knowledge of them it is altogether impossible to think fruitfully about the social question.

Now let us ask ourselves (we have often touched upon this question, but today we will bring out certain other details) what is the fundamental quality of soul, the fundamental and decisive quality which is brought out in the age that began in the fifteenth century and that will last, as I told you, on into the third millennium. This fundamental quality, which has scarcely yet shown itself in its true form but only in its first beginning and which is evolving and will evolve ever more and more, is that of human intelligence, intelligence as a property of the soul. Thus in the course of this age human beings will more and more be called upon to judge about all things out of their own intelligence and notably about social, scientific and religious matters, for indeed, the religious, the scientific and the social impulses do in a certain sense exhaustively describe the range of human life.

Now perhaps this conception of the intelligent human being, which we must necessarily awaken in ourselves, will be understood more easily if you realize the following. It cannot be said of the fourth post-Atlantean age[48] in the same sense as of the present time that the human being wished to establish his personality purely on the basis of the intelligence. I brought this out very clearly in my book *The Riddles of Philosophy* with regard to philosophical thinking. In the fourth post-Atlantean age, ending in the fifteenth century AD, it was not necessary for human beings to make use of their intelligence in a personal way. The concepts, the ideas, that is to say the intelligent element, flowed into human beings with their perceptions of the environment, with their other relationships in life to the world, just as colours and sounds enter the human being in perception. Notably for the Greeks, the intellectual content was a perception; and it was so also for the Romans.

For the human beings of modern times, since the fifteenth century, the outcome of intellectual activity can no longer be a perception. The intellectual element is excluded from the world of perceptions. Human beings no longer receive concepts and ideas at one and the same time with perceptions. It is wholly an error to imagine that this great change did not take place at the turn of the fifteenth century. This kind of error, this inability to make distinctions, has indeed been perceived by some people even in ordinary outer life. Thus a European, as we can easily realize, is apt to see all Japanese exactly alike. Although they are just as different from one another as Europeans are, yet he does not distinguish them. So, too, modern learning does not distinguish between the several epochs, but imagines them all alike. But that is not the case. On the contrary, a mighty change took place, for instance, at the turn of the fifteenth century when human beings ceased to perceive the concepts at one and the same time with perception, when they began really to have to work out their concepts. For human beings of the present day have to work out concepts out of their own person- alities. We are only in the initial stages of it. It will become more and more so.

Now the human beings of the west, the middle and the east are in the highest degree differentiated, especially with regard to this development of the intelligence. And since the theoretical demands of the proletariat today — as is natural in the fifth post-Atlantean age, the age of the spiritual soul — are brought forward as intelligent demands, it is necessary to consider the relationships and differentiations of the intelligent nature of the human soul across the earth also in relation to the social impulses.

The significance of these things is underestimated because they still work today so largely in the sub- conscious. Human beings with their lazy thinking are not anxious to make clear distinctions in clear consciousness. But every human being has an inner human being within him raying forth into his consciousness only to a certain extent. And this inner human being makes very clear and sharp distinctions, distinctions for example as between western human beings, middle human beings and the eastern human beings according to their point of view, according as to whether they themselves are western, middle or eastern human beings.

I am not now referring to the single individuality as such, I mean what in human beings belongs to their nationality. I beg you always to observe this distinction. Of course the single individual rises out of the national element. Of course there are human beings today in whom the national element works scarcely at all. There are those who systematically try to be pure human beings without letting the national quality determine them. But to the extent that it does work in them it comes to expression in the varied ways which we have already characterized in these lectures. Today we will consider it once more from certain points of view and in relation to the social question.

In effect, whenever the social question emerges, when anything emerges that depends not only on the individual human being but on the community, the qualities of the nation, folk or people will always come into account. The member, let us say, of the British nation or the member of the German people or the person inhabiting Russian soil (I purposely distinguish them just in this way) may well have just the same views. But English, German and Russian policy or the social structures cannot be the same. They must be differentiated, for here the community comes into account. We are, therefore, calling into question not so much the individual relationship of human being to human being, but that which works from people to people, or differentiates the one nation from another. Again and again I must sharply emphasize this fact, for partly with good intentions and partly out of malice these things which I bring forward are repeatedly misunderstood.

Take one thing for example. I beg you to take these things *sine ira* quite objectively. They are not meant as criticizing but only as an indication of the facts. I beg you therefore to take them without any sympathies or antipathies. Let us consider a human being of Central Europe who observes the life of the English-speaking people and on the other side the life of the Russian-speaking people. He observes them as they come to expression in the characteristic ways of thinking of these peoples — once more then, not of the individual human beings but of the peoples as such.

Consciously, the Central European may pass all kinds of judgements. Needless to say, human beings today will say this or that according to public opinion, which is always equivalent to private laziness. That may be so, but the inner human being, the inner Central European human being, looking to the West, to the English-speaking people, and contemplating the nation as it expresses itself politically and socially will always pass the judgement, 'Philistines!' — though he need not bring it to consciousness at all. And when he looks across to Russia he will say

'Bohemians!' Of course that is somewhat radically spoken. And he himself will hear from left and right the answer: 'You may call us philistines, you may call us Bohemians, but you are a pedant.' Certainly that may be so; and it is once again judging from another point of view. But these things are more of a reality than one imagines, and they must be derived from the very depths of human evolution.

Now the peculiar thing is this. Within the English-speaking population the intelligence is instinctive. It works instinctively. It is a new instinct that has arisen in the evolution of humankind — the instinct to think intelligently. The very thing the spiritual soul will have to educate, the intelligence, is practised instinctively by the English-speaking people. The English people have a native talent for the instinctive exercise of the intelligence.

The Russian people differ from the English as the North Pole does from the South (or I might even say as the North Pole does from the Equator) with respect to this impulse of the intelligent being in human beings. In Central Europe, as I have said before now, human beings do not have intelligence instinctively, they must be educated to it. Intelligence must be trained and developed in them. That is the tremendous difference. In England and America the intelligence is instinctive. It has all the qualities of an instinct. In Central Europe nothing of intelligence is born in a person. One must be trained, brought up to it. It must be grasped in the development of man. In Russia it is so, that people even argue with one another as to what the intelligence really is. I could refer to many instances of this in literature, you must not think that I construct these things myself.

According to many statements by Russians with real insight, what they call the intelligence is something quite different from what is called so in Central Europe, let alone in England. In Russia an intelligent person is not someone who has studied this and that. Whom do we call an intellectual here? We call 'intellectuals' those who have studied, who have made this or that subject their own, and have thus trained themselves in thinking. As I said, in Western Europe and America the intelligence is even a native quality, born in them. We shall certainly not go so far as to exclude from the intelligentsia the businessman, the civil servant, or a member of any one of the liberal professions. But the Russian will do so most decidedly. He will not consider a businessman, a civil servant, or a member of one of the liberal professions so easily a 'man of intelligence'. No, among the Russians a man of intelligence must be a man who is awake, who has attained a certain self-consciousness. The civil servant who has studied much, who even has a judgement on many things, need not be an enlightened person. But the worker who thinks about his connection with the social order, who is awake as to his relation to society, he is a man of intelligence. It is very indicative that in Russia one is obliged to apply the word intelligence in quite a different sense. For whereas in the West the intelligence is instinctive, born in one, and in the middle one is trained to it, or at any rate it is evolved in one, in the East it is treated as something that is certainly not born in one—nor can one merely be trained to it. It is not merely evolved, it is something that awakens from out of a certain depth within the human soul. Human beings awaken to intelligence. This fact has been observed especially by certain members of the Cadet Party who say that this faith in enlightenment or awakening is the very reason why a certain arrogance and conceit is to be found in the intelligentsia of Russia, despite all their other qualities of humility.

The fact is that this intelligence in Russia has a very special part to play in the evolution of humankind. If you do not let yourselves be deceived, if you do not give yourselves up to illusions of external symptoms, but go to the heart of the matter, then—however insignificant it appears to you in one or another Russian according to your Western or Central European ideas—you will recognize that this intelligence is being preserved and guarded from all instinctive qualities. Such indeed is the idea of the Russian; the intelligence must not be corrupted by any kind of human instinct, nor must we imagine that anything worth mentioning has been attained with all the intellectuality to which we train and educate ourselves. Russians—unconsciously, needless to say—want to preserve and keep the intelligence until the coming of the sixth post-Atlantean age, which is their age. So that when that time comes, they will not reach down with their intelligence into human instincts but carry it upward into the region where the Spirit Self will blossom forth.

Whereas the English-speaking people let the intelligence sink down into the instincts, the Russians want above all to preserve and protect it. They do not want to let it go down into the instincts, they want to nurse and cherish it, little as it may be today, so as to keep it for the coming epoch when the Spirit Self — the purely spiritual — will be permeated with it.

When we regard the matter thus in its foundations, my dear friends, then even the things we would criticize root and branch with unbiased judgement will appear as arising out of a certain necessity in human evolution.

As I said, Russians themselves — Russians with insight who characterize these things — discover quite rightly that the Russian intelligence has a twofold basis which lies inherent in its evolution. Namely, it has received the configuration, the character it has today through the fact that Russians who have evolved intelligence and who claim to be wide awake and enlightened have been suppressed by the power of the police and had to defend themselves to the point of martyrdom against the violence of the police. As I said, we may well condemn this; but we must also reach a clear and unclouded judgement. The specific character of this Russian intelligence, seeking to preserve itself for future spiritual impulses of mankind, is absolutely conditioned on the one hand by the police suppression to the point of martyrdom. And on the other hand, in a perfectly natural way — as Russian authors themselves bring out again and again — this Russian intelligence (just because it wants to preserve itself for future ages) is today a thing remote from the world. It does not easily come to grips with life. It is directed to quite other things than are immediately active in the world. We may say therefore that in this respect too the Russian life of soul is the very opposite of what we find in the English-speaking population. In the West, we may say, the intelligence is protected by the police, in the East it is challenged and persecuted by the police. One person may prefer the one, another may prefer the other alternative. The point here is simply to characterize the facts. In the West, as I said, the intelligence is protected, its peculiar character is meant to flow into the outer life; it has to be inherent everywhere in the social structure. In the West it is the proper thing for people to take part through their intelligence in the social structure and the like. In Russia, no matter whether it be the Tsar or Lenin, the intelligence is suppressed by the police, and will continue to be so for a long time to come. Indeed, perhaps the very nerve and strength of it lies in the fact that it is suppressed by the police. We can combine these things, my dear friends, in a pretty epigrammatic way, and yet correctly. One can say, for instance, that in Russia the intelligence is persecuted, in Central Europe it is tamed, and in the West it is born tame. If we make these divisions, this differentiation, then — strange as the words may sound — we are hitting the nail on the head. In England and America the intelligence is born tame with respect to the constitution, with respect to external politics, indeed, even with respect to the social structure. In Central Europe it is tamed. In the

East where it would like freely to run about it is persecuted.

These are the things that must be considered if we
would see realities instead of approaching them merely in
a chaotic way, which can never lead to any real insight.
Now the point is this. On the one hand human beings are
differentiated in this way, notably with regard to the
intelligence, inasmuch as the nation or a people is working
in them. They are differentiated as I have spoken about
often and in various directions and am speaking about
again from a certain point of view today. On the other
hand, while in the age of the spiritual soul this differentiation must be clearly seen, we must find at the same
time the possibility to transcend it. There are two ways to
transcend these things in real life — in the first place by
learning to know them. So long as we only declaim from
general abstract points of view that this or that is the true
social standpoint, so long as we have no knowledge of the
differentiations of humankind, all our talk is valueless.
Insight into these things, that is the one thing of importance. The other is that we should still be able in a certain
way to rise above these things with human consciousness
and experience. In practice we must expect the
differentiations. We must not imagine that people are the
same all over the world, or that the social question can be
solved in the same way all over the world. We must know
that the social question has to be solved in different ways.
Out of the impulses in the different peoples it is seeking to
solve itself in different ways.

But this, my dear friends, is only possible on a foundation such as is provided here by spiritual science. For if you have some more or less chaotic — or even harmonious and consistent — social idea, how can you apply it, my dear friends? You can only apply it one-sidedly. You may have the most beautiful ideas, capable of absolute proof, so that you cannot but believe that all human beings, all over the earth, are to be made happy and prosperous by their means. Indeed it is the very misfortune of our times that people generally have such an idea in mind. Who is there that thinks differently in our time when he confronts his audience and puts forward his political or social ideas, that social conditions should be ordered thus and thus throughout the world by means of ideas I have thought up so that the whole of humankind will prosper? This is the way people think today, and, indeed, on the basis of our present habits of thought, it is scarcely possible for them to think in any other way.

But if you take the social impulse derived from spiritual science, which I explained to you a short while ago, you will see it has quite a different character. In fact it breaks with this habit of thought of our time. I said the point is not to have some uniform social ideal but to investigate what is seeking to realize itself. Then I drew your attention to a threefold structure of social life which has hitherto been gathered up chaotically into the unitary structured state. Today you will always see one cabinet, one parliament. Indeed it seems an ideal for the people of today to gather everything together chaotically into a single parliament. But as I said, the reality of things is tending to hold apart what is here being concentrated into one. The spiritual life, including the judicial (I do not mean general administration but the administration of civil and criminal law), constitutes one element, the economic life a second one and the life that regulates the two constitutes the third — general administration, public security and the like. These three relate to one another as states do today. They should deal with one another through their representatives, ordering their mutual relationships, but in themselves they should enjoy independent sovereignty.

Let what I am saying be reviewed and criticized and utterly condemned. One will be criticizing not a theory but something that wants to become reality in the next 40 or 50 years. And this threefolding will make it possible to reckon once more with the differentiation of humankind. For if you only have a unitary state you must force it upon all humanity like putting the some coat on a small, medium and very tall person (size is referred here only for the sake of illustration, I do not mean to describe nations as great or small). But this threefold structure contains inherent universality. For the social structure of the West will take shape in such a way that administration, the constitution, the general regulation of public life, public security in the widest sense, will preponderate. The other two will be to some extent subordinate, dependent on this one. In other regions of the world it will be different again. Once again one of the three will predominate and the other two will be more or less subordinate. With a threefold conception you have the possibility to find, in your own view of things, the differentiation of realities. A unitary idea must be extended over the whole earth, but if a thing is inherently threefold you can say: in the West the one is predominant; in the middle the second is predominant; and in the East the third is predominant. Thus what you find as the ideal of the social structure will be differentiated over the whole of the earth. This is the fundamental difference of the view here presented out of spiritual science from other views. This view is applicable to realities from the very outset because it can be differentiated within itself and applied in a differentiated way to the realities of life. Such is the difference between an abstract and a concrete view of things. An abstract theory consists of so many concepts of which one believes that they will bring happiness. A concrete view is one of which one knows; its nature is such that something can grow and develop in the one case, something else in another, and a third in a different case again. The first or second or third will be applicable to the corresponding external conditions. This is what distinguishes a view of realities from all dogmatism. Dogmatism swears by dogmas, and dogmas can only maintain their sway by tyrannizing realities. A conception of reality is like the reality itself; it is inherently a living thing. Like the human or any other organism, it is mobile and alive, not fixed and rigid. In the same way a real conception inherently lives, grows or develops, now in one direction, now in another.

If we observe this difference in conception of reality and

dogmatism, it is very important in helping to change the habits of thought within the soul which people need so badly today and from which they are yet so far removed — far more so than they know. And what I am now telling you is connected profoundly with anthroposophical spiritual science. You see, for the ordinary science of today the human being himself is a single unit. The anatomist, the physiologist studies the brain, the sense organs, nerves, liver, spleen and heart. For him they are all organs placed in a single unitary organism. We do not do so. We distinguish the human being related to the head, or nerves and senses, from the human being related to the chest, or respiration and blood circulation, and, finally, the human being related to the metabolism, the extremities and muscles. We distinguish, as you know, the threefold human being existing in the world. And because we do not adhere abstractly to the onefold human being, anthroposophical spiritual science discovers the kind of social organism into which the human being as a threefold being fits. For the guiding thread is always the anthro-posophical structuring of the human being. After all, those three elements themselves are, more or less, the outer symbols of a person's being. For the person himself is rooted in all the worlds. We shall find in this threefold human being a guiding thread to understand in turn the differentiation of humankind across the world.

Now when I speak plainly about these things I would ask you once more to take them *sine ira*, for I am merely describing. I am not criticizing nor am I saying anything to detract from the one side or to find favour with the other side in any way. Let us begin with the Russian human being, the Eastern European human being. We simply cannot study him if we only bear in mind anatomy, physiology or psychology as it is today. We can only study him if we bear in mind the threefold human being whose nature I have indicated in broad outline in my book *The Riddles of the Soul*. For if we consider the specific characteristics of the Russian soul and the Russian people of today in general—please note: of today—then we shall have to say that in Russia (may our Russian friends forgive me, but it is true) the human being relating to the head is at home. I say that our Russian friends should forgive me for they themselves do not believe it. But they are wrong. They no doubt will say: the human being related to the heart is at home in Russia, and the head of all things is far less prominent. But you can only make such a statement if you do not study spiritual science properly. For the Russian head culture appears predominantly as a culture of the heart. Because—if I may put it tritely—the Russian has his heart in his head. That is to say, his heart works so strongly that it works up towards his head, crosses his whole intelligence, permeates everything. It is the working of the heart upon the head, upon the concepts and ideas, which configures the whole of Eastern European culture.

And once more, I hope that the Central European will not take offence, but it simply is so: their essential characteristic—and this describes the whole of Central European culture — is that their head is perpetually falling into their chest, while on the other hand the abdomen or the extremities are perpetually being drawn up into the heart. That is the essential thing in Central Europe. Hence it is so frightfully hard for him to find his bearings, for he is neither at the one end nor at the other. I described this when I said recently that in the Guardian of the Threshold[49] the Central European experiences above all a wavering, tottering uncertainty and doubt.

Once again, may our West European friends not be offended with me for — you are already anticipating what is left — their culture is essentially an abdominal, a muscular culture. That is their peculiarity — in the nation, not in the single individual as such. All that proceeds from the culture of the muscles works strongly even into the head. Hence the instinctive quality of their intelligence. Hence too it is there that we find the origin of muscular culture in the modern sense — sport and so forth. Indeed, you will find evidence of all that I am saying everywhere in external life if only you are willing and prepared to look at the facts objectively. Anthroposophical spiritual science will give you the guiding thread for this purpose. In the Russian it is so that his heart rises up into the head. In the English-speaking people the abdomen rises up into the head, but the head reacts in turn upon the lower body and directs it. It is very important to consider these things. We need not always express them so radically as we do amongst ourselves. After all, here we understand one another, we have a certain measure of good will towards one another. We know how to take these things objectively, not on the basis of sympathy and antipathy.

Thus you see, we must look at the threefold human being; we must really know that the human being is a threefold being, a being after the pattern of the Trinity, even when we are studying his physiological and psychological differentiations. And this is the essential thing; people must have an interest in one another not merely as the parson preaches it, but a real interest from person to person, which can after all only be founded on real insight. It remains an empty abstraction to say: 'I love all people.' To approach the other human beings with understanding is what is needed, and likewise it is necessary to approach the different human communities with understanding if one is to have a true judgement about them and about their social structure. And this can only be the case when one knows the threefold nature of the human being. Unless you know what is the predominant bodily feature in a community of human beings—please do not misinterpret what I am saying—you cannot really know them. To gain a real insight you must have some guiding thread, otherwise you will confuse and muddle things. That is the point. That is why anthroposophical spiritual science is a thing that takes reality into account. Hence it is a thing that people often find unpleasant, for as a result of certain prejudices people do not want to be seen through, not even in private life. They find it dreadfully unpleasant to be seen through. We might almost say that of any ten men, at least nine will be your enemies if you really see through them. In one way or another they will become your enemies. People do not like being seen through, even when it happens in the light that is communicated here, so that it may serve to enhance the love of humanity. For the abstract love of humanity (I have often used this comparison) is like the warmth that the stove ought to develop. You tell it: 'You are a stove. It is your duty as a stove to warm the room.' But if you do not stoke it, all your moral talk is useless. So it is with all the Sunday afternoon addresses. However much you preach love and love again, if you do not provide the fuel whereby human beings and communities of human beings are known and understood, all your preaching is worthless. Anthroposophical spiritual science is fuel to kindle the right interest from person to person—the real development of human love. Even the historical facts—I developed them here some time ago in symptomatic form—underlying the social impulses of today can only be brought home to human understanding from the standpoint of a conception of realities.

When we consider what we have already said of the differences between the Western, Middle and Eastern world, something that will flow into your souls still more abundantly if with its help you now observe these worlds with understanding, then perhaps we may ask: how is it— apart from what we have already said—that the Russian intelligence can preserve itself for a future time? It needs a greater strength to protect the intelligence from the encroaching instincts than it requires to exercise the native instinctive intelligence. It needs a greater strength. And this too has been attained by certain arrangements, if I may call them so, in the evolution of Western humanity. Take only this one instance that Russia has in many respects been held aloof from the cultural currents and movements that have taken their course in the West. I once described to you from another point of view this damming up, this congestion of a civilization of former ages towards the East. See for instance how the division of the Church took place in the ninth century and was completed in the tenth. An earlier form of Christianity was driven back towards the East, there to remain stationary and conservative. Thus we may say: a certain state which was spread over the whole of Christendom in early centuries has been driven eastwards and has there remained stationary. Meanwhile the West has continued to evolve it: Christianity. Thus something was pushed back towards the East. That on the one side. Meanwhile from eastward of the Russian East something was projected into the East, namely, the Tartar element and all that came from Asia. All this is only an expression of the fact that on the Russian soil earlier forces of humanity have been crowded back and have received into themselves the human forces that came from Asia in a more youthful state than West European humanity.

Or again, consider the Central European civilization in its dependence on Protestantism—a dependence far greater than is generally thought. At bottom, the whole civilization of Central Europe is configured out of the impulse of Protestantism. I do not mean this or that religious creed; I mean the impulse of Protestantism, for Protestantism itself is but a symptom for anyone regarding these things from a higher vantage point. The essential thing is the spiritual impulse working in it. Take the science and scholarship that is carried on in Central Europe; the whole form of its development is influenced by Protestantism. Without Protestantism Central European culture is utterly unthinkable.

Now what appears so predominantly at one place is present differently, in a different relationship to life, at another. It is as I illustrated just now when I spoke of the social tasks of anthroposophy which must be applied in differentiated ways. What has Protestantism been in Central Europe? One might say that Protestantism gave the first impetus to human beings supporting themselves on their own intelligent nature. The Central European intelligence, of which I said that it has to be trained and educated, is very closely connected with Protestantism. Even the Catholic action which arose against Protestantism is, rightly considered, Protestant in character except when it happens to proceed from the Jesuits, who have deliberately held back the impulse that came through Protestantism. This inner impulse, working through Protestantism, works, if I may put it so, in its purest essence in Central Europe. How did it work in Western Europe? Study the historic facts in the proper symptomatic way and you will find that the working of Protestantism in Western Europe and in America corresponds as a matter of course to the inborn intelligent instinct. Indeed it comes to expression more in the political than in the religious life. It works as a perfect matter of course. It permeates everything. It does not need a special statement or constitution. Albeit here and there reformist hearts were kindled into flame, it does not need to bring forth so shattering a Reformation as took place in Central Europe. In the West it exists as a matter of course. At this point we might even say that modern Western human beings are born as Protestants. The Central European discusses and argues as a Protestant. In Central Europe, Protestantism above all provokes discussions about the things of intelligence. Here it is not inborn. And Russians — as Russians — absolutely reject Protestantism; they will have nothing to do with it. Indeed, as Russians they simply will not have it. Russian culture and Protestantism are incompatible.

What I am now saying comes to expression not only in the religious confessions but in the reception of any kind of cultural impulse. Take Marxism for example. You can trace its course in the Western countries. There it is received from the very outset as a straightforward protest against the old conditions with regard to property and the like. In the Central Powers there is much discussion on those things and much argument and bickering and doubt, and much useless talk. All this arises out of the character of the Central Powers. And in Eastern Europe Marxism takes on the strangest forms. There it must first be completely transformed. Take the Marxism of Eastern

Europe; you will find it permeated, tinged through and through by the spirit of Russian Orthodoxy—not in its ideas, but in the way the Russian relates himself to it. Marxism in Russia bears the stamp of Orthodox faith.

All this is only to draw your attention to the need to look beyond the externals and see the true inward character of things. Much will be gained if you become accustomed to telling yourself in relation to many things in life that words as they are used today are to a great extent devalued coinage. That people think according to the customary usage of words is never really in accordance with reality — we must look deeper everywhere. Protestantism, for instance, defined in the usual way according to present-day habits of thought no longer expresses a reality. We must conceive of it in such a way as to recognize how it appears in Marxism, or in politics generally, or even in science. Then we shall have something that accords with the reality. So radically is it necessary for us to strive to get beyond the mere semblances of words and concepts, and to take hold of real life. Everything depends on this, and on this above all depends the right conception of the most important impulse of the present time, which is the social impulse. On this depends a true judgement of the facts of our time. It is precisely because people are so unaccustomed to look at reality, because people are far removed from thoughts that are in tune with reality, that current circumstances are so misjudged. They always raise questions about guilt or innocence in the most recent military catastrophes although the question as such is completely irrelevant. That is why I spoke to you here some time ago about the true state of affairs with regard to world impulses. Just as the map which I drew for you here is today being realized, other things are also being realized.[50] They are being realized and will do so just as they have been discussed here. One must develop a sense of what is really happening and not cling to the empty shells of words. Shells of words must often be used to characterize something but one should not become too attached to them. In the same way, if one perceives reality one must also understand from the perspective of reality the judgement today formed by the Entente and the Americans about the Central Powers. I have already said that when this catastrophe of the war began I heard many people severely criticize what the Central European countries had done. What is now happening to a much greater extent is a policy of force and so one is criticized much less today by those who criticized previously although there is enough cause for harsh criticism. I believe that I have never spoken in defence of certain persons but only described circumstances. Hence it cannot be seen as my task, either, to defend personalities in any way whose real existence has been exposed recently. But whether the complete adoration of Wilsonism for example and everything associated with it is less founded in people's tendency to some kind of idolatry than what developed in the Central Powers as worship of Ludendorff, a clear case of social insanity, is an issue which must be considered very carefully, which cannot be decided superficially.

I once told you here from a different perspective that when one person is angry with another and says harsh things, the cause is not always—indeed in the rarest cases—to be found in the other person. The latter may of course be bad; but this badness is the least reason for the anger, as anyone who observes reality objectively can see. No, for the most part the cause of the anger is a need to be angry. And this need to be angry seeks an object, it needs to be released. And it seeks to bring its thoughts into such a form that they appear to be justified in the soul of the angry person. That is how it often is in the relationship of individuals with one another. But in the large affairs of the world it is no different; only here we must bear in mind that there are also deeper reasons. You see, it is perfectly intelligible and natural for people in the Entente and American countries now to criticize and condemn root and branch not only individual leaders but the whole population of the Central Powers, and to say all manner of things in this direction. We can well understand it, for what would the policy of the Entente countries in these weeks look like if the people in those countries were to say: the people in the Central Powers are not so bad after all, at bottom they are only human beings, they need only develop the better aspects of their nature, then they are quite all right. Indeed, if they were to say that, it would agree very badly with the policy they are now pursuing. In the world, one must say the things that justify one's action.

We must know how things proceed on the basis of reality. That is a deeper way of seeing things. It goes without saying that the entire public opinion of the Entente countries is as it is not because it is true but in order to justify their own attitude. Just as it often happens when a person gets angry with another, he does so not because the person he is angry with is like this or like that, but because he has a need to be angry about something and wants to let it out. It really is necessary to see things differently from the way we are used to seeing them. And this is the whole point: understanding spiritual science in the inmost foundations of one's soul is in many respects a very different thing from what is conceived even by many who call themselves adherents of the anthroposophical movement.

Outwardly, abstractly considered — and here we come to a different chapter — one might believe that the social-ism, the social demands of the present day proceed from social impulses. I described the other day how man oscillates between social and antisocial impulses or instincts. An abstract thinker would take it as a matter of course that the socialist member of the proletariat of the present time is a product of social impulses. For it is proper, is it not, to define the social by the social. But it is not true. Anyone who considers the socialism of the pro-letariat of the present day in its reality knows well that socialism as it appears in the Marxism of today is an antisocial phenomenon, a product of antisocial impulses. Such is the difference between abstract definition, abstract thinking and realistic thinking. Ask yourselves: what is the driving force in those who are seeking to realize socialism in the direction to which I am referring? Are they being driven by social instincts? No, by antisocial instincts. I even demonstrated that yesterday on the basis of external characteristics, on the basis of the configuration of the formula 'Workers of the world unite!' That is to say; 'Feel hatred against other classes in order that you may feel the bond that unites you.' There you have one of the antisocial impulses. And we might adduce very many antisocial impulses if we studied the social psychology of the present day. Such is the difference between the way of thought that is arising and evolving — that must arise and evolve and that is to be helped on by spiritual science — and all that lies in the current thinking habits of today.

Hence, too, the anthroposophical standpoint which must be put forward in relation to the social question meets as yet with so much opposition. For people cannot think in accordance with realities. Above all, they cannot think in a differentiated way; and if anyone does think in this way, it is frequently thought that this person is contradicting himself.

Important issues of the present day will only be solved by realistic thinking. I will tell you one such issue relating to what we have already spoken of. I said that the thing that is rumbling especially in the minds of the proletariat and that constitutes a motivating force in them is this: the ancient slave has been replaced by the modern enslavement of labour inasmuch as in the present social structure labour is a commodity. Indeed, the threefold social structure of which I have told you already contains the impulse to separate the commodity from human labour. For the effect of this threefold order is not logical conclusions but conclusions in reality which also correspond to the reality of what we perceive.

Now this question is followed by another, an absolutely burning question at the present moment. One of the fundamental demands of the materialism of the proletariat with its Marxist colouring is the nationalization of the means of production. The means of production are to be given over to common ownership and this would only represent the first move towards common ownership of property in general, of land and so forth. It is a part of the programme of the Russian Soviet Republic, which I explained to you, to nationalize, or better said, socialize the means of production and the land. This in turn points to the most important subsidiary social question of the present. This can be formulated as follows: is social action in our current culture, or, indeed, the current chaos if we consider the Central Powers and the countries of the East, to happen in such a way that there is a trend towards individuals becoming owners or should the development be such that the community becomes the owner? You understand what I mean — should it be the individual who has ownership or should those things which can be owned, such as land, means of production and so on, become communal property to avoid injustice? That is a very important subsidiary social question. Today the tendency of proletarian thinking is to make things communal property. But for the most important social impulses, it makes no difference at all whether an individual or an association or the community as such is the owner. To anyone who is able to study the realities, this is clearly revealed. In relation to the individual worker the community will be no different from, no less bad as an employer than an individual entrepreneur. This lies in the nature of the case, it is like a law of nature; people only fail to see it, and hence they are misled. For the real question is this: should all people become owners of property? That would happen if, instead of having communal property (I cannot here explain the technique, but it is perfectly feasible), the individuals—every one of them—owned property in a just way according to the given opportunities in any territory. Should everyone become a property owner or should everyone join the proletariat? That is the alternative. The present thinking of the proletariat wants to make everyone join the proletariat so that the community alone would be entrepreneur. But if we can see the reality, the very opposite will be the outcome. The threefold nature of the social structure can never be attained by making everyone into the proletariat. The tendency of the threefold structure must really be to attain the freedom of the individual in respect of body, soul and spirit. That will not to be attained by everyone joining the proletariat, but it will be achieved for every individual if everyone possess a certain basis of property.

The second thing that must be achieved is a regulation of social conditions, such that before the law or constitution, before the government in fact, everyone is equal:

liberty in spiritual matters; equality in the state if that is what people want to continue calling this third; and fraternity in relation to the economic life. I know well-written books which rightly emphasize that the three ideals of liberty, equality and fraternity contradict one another. It is true, equality decidedly contradicts liberty. Clever writers said this even in 1848 or even earlier. If we muddle everything together these things contradict one another. There must be liberty in the spiritual and judicial domain, the domain of religion, education and juris-prudence. There must be equality in administration, the government and public security. There must be fraternity in the economic domain. In the economic domain we have property which must be developed for the future. In the domain of public security and administration we must have right and in the domain of spiritual life and juris-prudence we must have liberty. When divided into a trinity, these things are not in contradiction with one another. For here the things that contradict one another in thought do not do so in reality because in reality they are distributed to the different domains. The mere thought burrows for contradictions; but the reality lives in con-tradictions. We cannot grasp the reality, if we cannot grasp the contradictions and deal with them in our thinking. So you see, spiritual science as here intended certainly has something to say on the most important questions of our time. Perhaps a few of you will yet realize this fact, and realize moreover that the whole way we think about this spiritual science of anthroposophy should be influenced by the awareness of its relation to the most important requirements of our time.

This indeed is closely connected with the way in which I personally, for instance, imagine how anthroposophically oriented spiritual science and its carrier, the anthro- posophically-oriented movement, should take its stand in the spiritual life of our time. Of course it cannot be achieved all at once that our contemporaries should see these things in the right way. Do not believe — and anyone who knows me will certainly not believe this — that I say these things out of any personal foolishness or vanity. But I am compelled again and again by the facts to char- acterize what happens in one direction or another. It is truly the case — and I have demonstrated it to you on many an occasion — that I myself am not at all inclined to over- estimate what I can do and claim to do. I know my limi- tations and am well aware of many things of which a number of people may have no idea that I am aware of. But for those who to some extent can judge me rightly in this direction, I may perhaps say how much I would wish — the expression is not quite right but there is no other — something to happen. It is this, my dear friends, that there should be a certain sense of discrimination between what is intended here, and other things with which it is so frequently confused. There are still so many people today, who, seeing here or there this or that occult society or society that calls itself occult, will not distin- guish it as healthy human understanding can distinguish it from what is to be found here. For, imperfect as it may be, here there is at least the real striving to take the consciousness of the age into account. Look on the other hand at all the other things that are frequently considered as occult or similar movements. How do they take the consciousness of the time into account? Look at all the Masons of low and high degrees, look at all the different religious communities; it is precisely the antiquated thing about them that they are unable really to reckon with the consciousness of our time. Where else do we find people speaking on a solid basis? Where do we find them speaking out on the burning questions of the time in a way that really enters into modern life, that is adapted to the realities? You will not be able to discover these things in any of the rituals and instructions of this or that Masonic or religious community. This is what I would desire—a real sense of discrimination.

I admit that this is made more difficult because owing to historical circumstances that I once described to you this Society was confused in the beginning with the Theosophical Society or all manner of other societies.[51] Outwardly considered, it may have been a mistake; karmically it was justified. It would have been cleverer if this Anthroposophical Society, standing entirely independently, had been founded without any relation to other societies. Outwardly conceived, it would certainly have been more wise. For all the philistinism, the bourgeois characteristics of the Theosophical Society and all the antiquated stuff would not have flowed into it. Not that it has flowed into anthroposophy—it has not. But it has entered into the life and habits of the society. If only anthroposophy lived rightly in our society — which it does not — this society could, in a certain sense at least, be a perfect example to characterize one third of the social structure which flows from anthroposophy itself. I mean the spiritual third, including the juridical sphere. For what should apply between individuals among anthroposophists as the sphere of rights should really go without saying. I always feel it to be the sharpest and bitterest breach with the spirit which should develop among us when one member speaks of another in such a way that he goes outside to complain or to accuse. Here too the consciousness of rights should develop, in so far as it is included in the one third of the social structure. But we have a long way to go yet to gain an Anthroposophical Society such as is really intended, containing what it might contain out of the impulses of anthroposophy. First of all we must evolve an ear for inner truth which so few people have today. Because this sense of discrimination which should really come from without fails so to come. It is necessary for me now and then to point to the distinctive features from one point of view or another. And today, especially with regard to certain things, I would say this: what lives through me in the anthroposophical movement is distinguished from other things in one essential respect. I have always worked according to the principle which I stated in the preface to the first edition of my *Theosophy*, namely, that I communicate nothing other than what I can communicate from my own personal experience. I communicate nothing other than what I can stand for from my own personal experience. Here at this place there is no appealing to authorities such as is cultivated so much in other quarters.

This has certain consequences. I may truly say that the spiritual stream which is guided through the anthroposophical movement depends upon no other stream. It depends alone on the spirituality that is flowing through the present time. Hence I am under no obligation—I ask you to take this in all earnestness—I am under obligation to no one to keep silent about anything of which I myself consider that it ought to be spoken about in our time. There is no rule of silence for a person who is obliged to no one for his spiritual treasure—there is no rule of silence.

That will already give you a basis for distinguishing this movement from others. For if anyone should ever say that that which is proclaimed in anthroposophical spiritual science is proclaimed in any other way than in the sense of what was said in my *Theosophy*, namely, that I myself am answerable for it purely out of my own experience, if anyone should ever say this, then he may not know the facts, or he has frequently been absent, or he has only seen them from outside. But whether it be from malice or otherwise, he is proclaiming an untruth. But someone, on the other hand, who has frequently been with us and says something else, let us say he alleges some 'past' or a connection of this spiritual movement with another, knowing all the time the facts and circumstances here among us—he is telling lies. That is the point, my dear friends. He will either be telling an untruth through ignorance of the facts, or, knowing the facts well, he will be lying. That is how all the opponents to this movement must be seen.

Hence I must emphasize again and again: I have only to keep silence concerning those things of which I know that they cannot yet be communicated to humankind owing to its immaturity. But there is nothing on which I must keep silence in connection with anyone to whom any vow has been made, or for any such reason. Never has anything flowed into this movement that came from another side. Spiritually, this movement was never dependent on any other. The connections were always only of an external character. Perhaps the time will come when you will see that it is well to remember that I sometimes say things in advance which only afterwards become apparent in their right context. If you have the good will, the time may come when it will serve you well to remember the sense in which the spiritual treasure that must flow through the anthroposophical movement is being cultivated here.

Nevertheless, there is a touchstone for anyone who is willing to distinguish this anthroposophical movement from other movements. There is a touchstone available today for such a movement and it is threefold. First, such a movement must show itself equal to the scientific and intellectual requirements of the time. Go through all the literature that I have produced; however imperfect in this or that detail, you will see everywhere the earnest effort to create a movement drawing not on old antiquated sources but thoroughly at home in the scientific methods of the present time and working in full harmony with the present scientific consciousness. That is the one thing.

The second is this: that such a movement has something really essential to say on the vital questions of the present time — on the social question for instance. Try comparing what other movements have to say in this direction in their antiquated character, in their remoteness from reality, with what this movement has to say. The third part of the touchstone is this: that such a movement can consciously explain the different religious needs of humankind to themselves, can explain them and clarify them. That is to say, it combines enlightenment concerning the religious needs of humankind with a full and actual acquaintance with the realities.

Herein already you can distinguish this movement from all those which basically provide no more than Sunday afternoon sermons, which can well manage to sermonize on morality and the like but have no idea about the concrete concepts active in the present social structures. A science dealing with the realities of our time must be able to speak on labour, capital, credit, the land, about the things connected with life today, on the development of the social life, as easily as it can speak about the relation of human beings to the divine being, on loving thy neighbour and so forth. This is what humankind has omitted to do for so long — to find the real connections, from the highest realms down to the most immediate and concrete developments and processes of life. This is what theology and theosophy in their various forms in our time have left undone, and what a certain occult movement too has left undone. They talk from above downwards until they reach the point where they can tell people: be good people and so on. But they are unproductive, they are sterile when it comes to really grasping the burning issues of the time. External science and scholarship can speak of these immediate things of life, but they speak in a way that is remote from realities. I showed you yesterday how estranged they are from actual life. After all, how many people are there today who know what capital is, what it really is? True, they know when they have a certain amount of money in a safe that it is so much capital. But that is not knowing what capital is. To know what capital is, is to know how the social structure is regulated with respect to certain things and processes. Just as for the individual human being we must know anthroposophically the relationships that obtain in the blood circulation that rhythmically regulates human life, so we must know what is pulsating in the most varied ways in social life. But present-day physiology is not even able to solve the most important questions in materialistic terms for they can only be solved by anthroposophical insight into the threefold human being.

What, for instance, does present-day science know about one immensely important question, namely, what is the basis of our ideas, purely materialistically speaking, what does the will depend on, purely materialistically speaking, in a certain respect? I can speak about these things today because, as I said before on another point, I have investigated them for 30 to 35 years. The basis of ideas is that as part of the blood circulation human beings have carbon dioxide within themselves which has not yet been exhaled. When carbon dioxide, not yet exhaled, is circulating inside a person you have the material counterpart, the material correlate of thought. And when there is oxygen in a person, oxygen not yet converted into carbon dioxide, oxygen that is still on the way to transformation into carbon dioxide, there, in a certain sense, you have the material correlate of the will. Where oxygen pulsates in human beings, oxygen not yet entirely transformed and fulfilling certain functions, there the will is at work in material terms. And where inside the human body there is carbon dioxide, not quite processed to the point of exhalation, there we have the material foundation for thought. But as to how these two poles—the thought pole which we can also call the carbon dioxide pole, and the will pole which we can also call the oxygen pole—as to how they are regulated, only a science of reality can tell. Nowhere in the books of today will you find the kind of truth as I have just expressed. Because people do not train their thinking with respect to this type of reality, they also fail to train it with respect to what is required for human beings today with regard to the social structure. But this will have to come, it is a requirement of our time. The social question must be made to include the question of how human beings, as beings of soul and spirit, fit into the social structure.

All these things have not been done. Think how different it would be if in any establishment the individual workers were involved also in terms of soul and spirit in the whole process which the commodity they make undergoes in the world, if they understood how they stand within the social structure through the fact that they produce this specific commodity. But this can only be realized if there is real interest from person to person to such an extent that in the course of time there will be no true adult unable to master the most important social concepts in a real way. The time must come—this is a social requirement—when people will simply know what capital and credit, cash and cheques are in their real economic effects. These things can be understood, they are not difficult; they need only be approached in the right way by those who teach them. The time will come when every person knows these things just as everyone knows today that soup is eaten not with a fork but with a spoon. Anyone who ate his soup with a fork would be behaving ridiculously, would he not? That the person who is ignorant of the other things is behaving ridiculously, too, must also become general public opinion.

Then the most important impulse of the present time— the social impulse—will be placed on a very different foundation.

6. Culture, Law and Economy

'Culture, Law and Economy',[52] *was published in the newspaper* Soziale Zunkunft *in September 1919. At this time Steiner's efforts to stimulate a grassroots movement for the threefold social order in post-war Germany was at its zenith. The article gives an exceptionally clear short sketch of the idea. Particularly important are Steiner's comments on the role a truly free cultural life could play in the social organization of modern times. As we never have experienced this potential it is very hard for most people to form an idea of what it could mean.*

In the present social movement there is a great deal of talk about social institutions, but very little about social and antisocial human beings. Very little regard is paid to the 'social question' that arises when one considers that institutions in a community take their social or antisocial stamp from the people who run them. Socialist thinkers expect to see in the community's control of the means of production something that will satisfy the demands of a wide range of people. They take for granted that under communal control of the economy human relations will necessarily assume a social form as well. They have seen that the economic system along the lines of private capitalism has led to antisocial conditions. They believe that when this industrial system has disappeared the antisocial tendencies at work within it will also necessarily come to an end.

Undoubtedly, along with the modern private capitalist form of industrial economy there have arisen social evils—evils that embrace the widest range of social life. But is this in any way a proof that they are a necessary consequence of this industrial system? An industrial system can, in and of itself, do nothing beyond putting men into life situations that enable them to produce goods for themselves or for others in a more or less efficient manner. The modern industrial system has brought the means of production under the power of individual persons or groups. The achievements of technology were such that the best use could be made of them by a concentration of industrial and economic power. So long as this power is employed in the one field—the production of goods alone—its social effect is essentially different from what it is when this power oversteps its bounds and trespasses into the fields of law or culture. It is this trespassing into the other fields that, in the course of the last few centuries, has led to the social evils that the modern social movement is striving to abolish. He who possesses the means of production acquires economic power over others. This economic power has resulted in the capitalist allying himself with the powers of government, whereby he is able to procure other advantages in society, opposing those who are economically dependent on him—advantages which, even in a democratically constituted state, are in practice of a legal nature. This economic domination has led to a similar monopolization of the cultural life by those who held economic power.

The simplest thing would seem to be to get rid of this economic predominance of individuals, and thereby do away with their dominance in the spheres of rights and spiritual culture as well. One arrives at this 'simplicity' of social thought when one fails to remember that the combination of technological and economic activity afforded by modern life necessitates allowing the most fruitful possible development of individual initiative and personal talent within the business community. The form production must take under modern conditions makes this a necessity. The individual cannot bring his abilities to bear in a business if in his work and decision-making he is tied down to the will of the community. However dazzling the thought is of the individual producing not for himself but collectively for society, its justice within certain bounds should not hinder one from also recognizing the other truth — collectively, society is incapable of giving birth to economic schemes that can be realized through individuals in the most desirable way. Really practical thought, therefore, will not look to find the cure for social ills in a reshaping of economic life that would substitute communal production for private management of the means of production. Rather, the endeavour should be to forestall evils that may spring up along with management by individual initiative and personal talent without impairing this management itself. This is possible only if neither the legal relationship among those engaged in industry nor that which the spiritual-cultural sphere must contribute are influenced by the interests of industrial and economic life.

It cannot be said that those who manage the business of economic life can, while occupied by economic interests, preserve sound judgement on legal affairs and that, because their experience and work have made them well acquainted with the requirements of economic life, they will therefore be best able to settle legal matters that may arise within the workings of the economy. To hold such an opinion is to overlook the fact that a sphere of life calls forth interests arising only within that sphere. Out of the economic sphere one can develop only economic interests. If one is called out of this sphere to produce legal judgements as well, then these will merely be economic interests in disguise. Genuine political interests can only grow upon the field of political life, where the only consideration will be what are the rights of a matter. And if people proceed from such considerations to frame legal regulations, then the law thus made will have an effect upon economic life. It will then be unnecessary to place restrictions on the individual in respect of acquiring economic power; for such economic power will only result in his rendering economic services proportionate to his abilities — not in his using it to obtain special rights and privileges in social life.

An obvious objection is that political and legal questions do after all arise in people's dealings with one another in business, so it is quite impossible to conceive of them as something distinct from economic life. Theoretically this is right enough, but it does not necessarily follow that in practice economic interests should be paramount in determining these legal relations. The manager who directs a business must necessarily have a legal relationship to manual workers in the same business; but this does not mean that he, as a business manager, is to have a say in determining what that relationship is to be. Yet he will have a say in it, and he will throw his economic predominance into the scales if economic cooperation and legal administration are conjoined. Only when laws are made in a field where business considerations cannot in any way come into question, and where business cannot gain any power over this legal system, will the two be able to work together in such a way that our sense of justice will not be violated, nor business acumen be turned into a curse instead of a blessing for the whole community.

When the economically powerful are in a position to use that power to wrest legal privileges for themselves, a corresponding opposition to these privileges will grow among the economically weak. As soon as it has become strong enough, such opposition will lead to revolutionary disturbances. If the existence of a separate political and legal province makes it impossible for such privileges to arise, then disturbances of this sort cannot occur. What this special legal province does is to give constant orderly scope to those forces which, in its absence, accumulate until at last they vent themselves violently. Whoever wants to avoid revolutions should learn to establish a social order that shall accomplish in the steady flow of time what will otherwise try to realize itself in one historical moment.

It will be said that the immediate concern of the modern social movement is not legal relations, but rather the removal of economic inequalities. One must reply to such an objection that our conscious thoughts are not always the true expression of the real demands stirring within us. Our conscious thoughts are the outcome of immediate experience, but the demands themselves originate in far deeper strata that are not experienced immediately. And if one aims at bringing about conditions that can satisfy these demands, one must attempt to penetrate to these deeper strata. A consideration of the relations that have come about in modern times between industrial economy and law shows that the legal sphere has become dependent upon the economic. If one were to try superficially, by means of a one-sided alteration in the forms of economic life, to abolish those economic inequalities that the law's dependence on the economy has brought about, then in a very short while similar inequalities would inevitably result as long as the new economic order were again allowed to build up the system of rights out of itself. One will never really touch what is working its way up through the social movement to the surface of modern life until one brings about social conditions in which, alongside the claims and interests of the economic life, those of politics and law can be realized and satisfied upon their own independent basis.

It is in a similar manner, again, that one must approach the question of the cultural life and its bearings on that of law and the economy. In the last few centuries the cultural life has been cultivated under conditions that allowed it to exercise only the smallest independent influence upon politics or the economy. One of the most important aspects of culture, education, was shaped by governmental interests. People were trained and taught according to the requirements of the state. And the power of the state was reinforced by economic power. If anyone were to develop his or her human capacities within the existing educational institutions, this depended directly on his or her economic station in life. Accordingly, the spiritual forces that were able to find scope within the political or economic spheres bore the stamp of these economic factors. Free cultural life had to forego any attempt to make itself useful within the political state. And it could influence the economic sphere only to the extent that economics had remained independent of state control. For a vibrant economy demands that competent people be given full scope; economic matters cannot be left to just anyone whom circumstances may have left in control. If, however, the typical socialist programme were to be carried out, and economic life were to be administered on the model of politics and the law, the cultivation of the free spiritual life would be forced to withdraw from the public sector altogether. However, a cultural life that has to develop apart from civil and economic realities loses touch with real life. It is forced to draw its substance from sources not vitally linked to those realities. Over the course of time the cultural life makes of this substance a sort of animated abstraction that runs alongside real events without having any concrete effect upon them. In this way, two different currents arise within cultural life. One of them draws its waters from political rights and economics, and is occupied with their daily requirements, trying to devise systems to meet these requirements— without, however, penetrating to the needs of our spiritual nature. All it does is devise external systems and harness men into them, ignoring what their inner nature has to say about it. The outer current of cultural life proceeds from the inner striving for knowledge and from ideals of the will. These it shapes to suit our inner nature. However, such knowledge is derived from contemplation; it is not the precipitate of practical experience. These ideals have arisen from concepts of what is true and good and beautiful, but they do not have the strength to shape the conduct of life. Consider what concepts, what religious ideals, what artistic interests, form the inner life of the shopkeeper, the manufacturer or the government official, outside and apart from his daily practical life; and then consider what ideas are contained in those activities that find expression in his bookkeeping, or for which he is trained by the education that prepared him for his profession. A gulf lies between these two currents of cultural life. The gulf has grown all the wider in recent years because the kind of thinking that is quite justified in natural science has become the measure of our relationship to reality as a whole. This way of thinking seeks to understand the lawfulness of phenomena that lie beyond human activity and human influence, so that the human being is a mere spectator of what he comprehends in a scheme of natural law. And although he sets these laws of nature into motion in technology, he himself does no more than allow the forces that lie outside his own being and nature to be active. The knowledge he employs in this kind of activity has a character that is quite different from his own nature. It reveals to him nothing of what lies in cosmic processes with which human nature is interwoven. For such knowledge as this he needs a world view that unites both the human world and the world outside him.

Anthroposophy strives for such knowledge. While fully recognizing all that scientific thinking means for the progress of modern humanity, anthroposophy sees that the scientific method framed for the study of nature is able to convey only that which comprehends the outer human being. It also recognizes the essential nature of the religious world views, but is aware that in the modern age these concepts of the world have become an internal concern of the soul, and not something applied in any way to the transformation of external life, which runs on separately alongside.

In order to arrive at its insights, spiritual science makes demands to which people are still little inclined because in the last few centuries they have become used to carrying on their outer and inner lives as two separate and distinct existences. Thus the incredulity that meets every endeavour to bring spiritual insight to bear upon social questions. People remember past attempts that were born of a spirit estranged from life. When there is any talk of such things, they recall Saint-Simon, Fourier, and others. The opinion is justified in so far as such ideas stem not from living experience, but rather from an artificial thought-construct. Thus they conclude that spiritual thinking is generally unable to produce ideas that can be realized in practical life. From this general theory come the various views that in their modern form are all more or less attributable to Marx. Those who hold them have no use for ideas as active agents in bringing about satisfactory social conditions. Rather, they maintain that the evolution of economic realities is tending inevitably towards a goal from which such conditions will result. They are inclined to let practical life more or less take its own course because in actual practice ideas are powerless. They have lost faith in the strength of spiritual life. They do not believe that there can be any kind of spiritual life able to overcome the remoteness and unreality that has characterized it during the last few centuries.

It is a kind of spiritual life such as this, nevertheless, that is the goal of anthroposophy. The sources it would draw from are the sources of reality itself. Those forces that hold sway in our innermost being are the same forces that are at work in external reality. Scientific thinking cannot penetrate down to these forces when it merely elaborates natural law intellectually out of external experience. Yet the world views that are founded on a more religious basis are no longer in touch with these forces either. They accept the traditions that have been handed down without penetrating to their fountainhead in the depths of human nature. The spiritual science of anthroposophy, however, seeks to penetrate to this fountainhead. It develops epistemological methods that lead down into those regions of our inner nature where the processes external to us find their continuation within human nature itself. The insights of spiritual science represent a reality actually experienced within our inmost self. These insights shape themselves into ideas that are not mere mental constructs, but rather something saturated with the forces of reality. Hence such ideas are able to carry within them the force of reality when they offer themselves as guides to social action. One can well understand that, at first, a spiritual science such as this should meet with mistrust. Such mistrust will not last when people come to recognize the essential difference that exists between this spiritual science and modern natural science, which is assumed today to be the only kind of science possible. If one can struggle through to a recognition of the difference, then one will cease to believe that one must avoid social ideas when one is intent upon the practical work of shaping social reality. One will begin to see, instead, that practical social ideas can be had only from a spiritual life that can find its way to the roots of human nature. One will see clearly that in modern times social events have fallen into disorder because people have tried to master them with thoughts from which reality constantly struggled free.

Spiritual insight that penetrates to the essence of human nature finds there motives for action that are immediately good in the ethical sense as well. The impulse towards evil arises in us only because in our thoughts and feelings we silence the depths of our nature. Accordingly, social ideas that are arrived at through the sort of spiritual concepts indicated here must, by their very nature, be ethical ideas as well. Since they are drawn not from thought alone, but from life, they possess the strength to take hold of the will and to live on in action. In true spiritual insight, social thought and ethical thought become one. And the life that grows out of such spiritual insight is intimately linked with every form of activity in human life—even in our practical dealings with the most insignificant matters. Thus as a consequence of social awareness, ethical impulse and practical conduct become so closely interwoven that they form a unity.

This kind of spirituality can thrive, however, only when its growth is completely independent of all authority except that derived directly from cultural life itself. Political and legal measures for the nurture of the spirit sap the strength of cultural life, while a cultural life that is left entirely to its own inherent interests and impulses will strengthen every aspect of social life. It is frequently objected that humanity would need to be completely transformed before one could found social behaviour upon ethical impulses. Such an objection does not take into account that human ethical impulses wither away if they are not allowed to arise within a free cultural life, but are instead forced to take the particular turn that the political-legal structure of society finds necessary for carrying on work in the spheres it has previously mapped out. A person brought up and educated within a free cultural life will certainly, through his very initiative, bring along into his calling much of the stamp of his or her own personality. Such a person will not allow himself to be fitted into the social machinery like a cog into a machine. In the end, however, what he brings into it will not disturb the harmony of the whole, but rather increase it. What goes on in each particular part of the communal life will be the outcome of what lives in the spirits of the people at work there.

People whose souls breathe the atmosphere created by a spirit such as this will vitalize the institutions needed for practical economic purposes in such a way that social needs, too, will be satisfied. Institutions devised to satisfy these social needs will never work so long as people feel their inner nature to be out of harmony with their outward occupation. For institutions of themselves cannot work socially. To work socially requires socially attuned human beings working within an ordered legal system created by a living interest in this legal system, and with an economic life that produces in the most efficient fashion the goods required for actual needs.

If the life of culture is a free one, evolved only from

those impulses that reside within itself, then legal institutions will thrive to the degree that people are educated intelligently in the ordering of their legal relations and rights; the basis of this intelligence must be a living experience of the spirit. Then economic life will be fruitful as well to the degree that cultivation of the spirit has developed new capacities within us.

Every institution that has arisen within communal life had its origin in the will that shaped it; the life of the spirit has contributed to its growth. Only when life becomes complicated, as it has under modern technical methods of production, does the will that dwells in thought lose touch with social reality. The latter then pursues its own course mechanically. We withdraw in spirit, and seek in some remote corner the spiritual substance needed to satisfy our souls.

It is this mechanical course of events, over which the individual will had no control, that gave rise to conditions which the modern social movement aims at changing. It is because the spirit that is at work within the legal sphere and the economy is no longer one through which the individual spiritual life can flow that the individual sees himself in a social order which gives him, as an individual, no legal or economic scope for self-development.

People who do not see through this will always object to viewing the social organism as consisting of three spheres, each requiring its own distinct basis — cultural life, political institutions and the economy. They will protest that such a differentiation will destroy the necessary unity of communal life. To this one must reply that right now this unity is destroying itself in the effort to maintain itself intact. Legal institutions based upon economic power actually work to undermine that economic power, because it is felt by those economically inferior to be a foreign body within the social organism.

And when the spirit that reigns within legal and economic life tries to regulate the activity of the organism as a whole, it condemns the living spirit (which works its way up from the depths of each individual soul) to powerlessness in the face of practical life. If, however, the legal system grows up on independent ground out of the consciousness of rights, and if the will of the individual dwelling in the spirit is developed in a free cultural life, then the legal system, strength of spirit and economic activity work together as a unity. They will be able to do so when they can develop, each according to its own proper nature, in distinct fields of life. It is just in separation that they will turn to unity; when an artificial unity is imposed, they become estranged.

Many socialist thinkers will thus dismiss such a view: 'It is impossible to bring about satisfactory conditions through this organic formation of society. It can be done only through a suitable economic organization.' They overlook the fact that those who work in their economic organization are endowed with wills. If one tells them this, they will smile, for they regard it as self-evident. Yet their thoughts are busy constructing a social edifice in which this 'self-evident fact' is ignored. Their economic organization is to be controlled by a communal will. However, this must after all be the result of the individual wills of the people united in the organization. These individual wills can never take effect if the communal will is derived entirely from the idea of economic organization. Individual wills can expand unfettered if, alongside the economic sphere, there is a legal sphere where the standard is set, not by any economic point of view but only by the consciousness of rights, and if, alongside both the economic and legal spheres, a free cultural life can find its place following only the impulses of the spirit. Then we shall not have a social order running like clockwork, in which individual will could never find a lasting place. Human beings will find it possible to give their wills a social bent and to bring them constantly to bear on the shaping of social circumstances. Under the free cultural life the individual will shall become social. When legal institutions are self-subsisting, these socially attuned individual wills shall yield a communal will that works justly. The individual wills, socially oriented and organized by the independent legal system, will exert themselves within the economic system, producing and distributing goods as social needs demand.

Most people today still lack faith in the possibility of establishing a social order based on individual wills. They have no faith in it because such a faith cannot come from a cultural life that has developed in dependence on the state and the economy. The kind of spirit that does not develop in freedom out of the life of the spirit itself but rather out of an external organization simply does not know what are the spirit's potentials. It looks about for something to guide and manage it, not knowing how the spirit guides and manages itself if it can but draw its strength from its own sources. It would like to have a board of management for the spirit — a branch of the economic and legal organizations — totally disregarding the fact that the economy and the legal system can thrive only when permeated with the spirit that is self-subsistent.

It is not good will that is needed in order to transform the social order; what is needed is courage to oppose this lack of faith in the spirit's power. A truly spiritual view can inspire this courage for such a spiritual view feels able to bring forth ideas that serve not only the inner needs of the soul, but also the needs of outer, practical life. The will to enter the depths of the spirit can become a will so strong as to suffuse every deed that one performs.

When one speaks of a spiritual view having its roots in life itself, many people take one to mean the sum total of those instincts that become a refuge when one travels along the familiar paths of life and holds every intervention from spiritual spheres to be a piece of eccentric idealism. The spiritual view intended here, however, must not be confused with that abstract spirituality incapable of extending its interests to practical life, nor with that spiritual tendency which actually denies the spirit flatly when it considers the orientation of practical life. Both these views ignore the way in which the spirit rules in the facts of external life, and therefore feel no urgent need to penetrate to its foundations. Yet only such a sense of urgency brings forth that knowledge which sees the 'social question' in its true light. The experiments now being made to resolve this issue yield such unsatisfactory results because many people have not yet become able to see the true nature of the question. They see this question arise in economic spheres, and they look to economic institutions to provide the answer. They think they will find the solution in economic transformation. They fail to recognize that these transformations can only come about through forces that are released from within human nature itself in the revival of an independent cultural and an independent legal life.

7. Central Europe between East and West

This is the first English publication of 'Central Europe between East and West'.[53] It is the text of a lecture Steiner delivered on the evening of 13 February 1921 in Stuttgart to a circle of people who were actively engaged in spreading the threefold idea in Central Europe at the time. It offers insights into the different perspectives and sentiments of peoples of the East, of the centre and of the West, ideas aimed at facilitating international cooperation at that time. It should be kept in mind that the Germany of the time was in danger of succumbing to communism, and social agitators of every ilk were active.

Looking at events currently taking place, you will see that all talk about social matters lacks any sort of foundation if it fails to take account of the international situation. That is why, for the purpose of the observations I wish to make here, I specifically chose the approach which has already become evident through our discussions of yesterday and today. I want to start by briefly setting out certain aspects of the international situation in order then to get on to our actual task on that basis.

The words I spoke earlier will have led you to ask what kind of thinking is required in order to come to a possible solution with regard to the great world historical issues of today and the foreseeable future. How should we think about the West on the one hand and the East on the other?

It is, after all, not difficult to see that there is a tendency today to think about everything in monolithic terms. A person wanting to form an opinion about the world situation today might think along the following lines with regard to a specific issue. From the West, we are faced with the prospect for the next decades of being subject to endeavours which want to force Central Europe to labour to support the West. And the only way to escape this threat is to adopt the same attitude — the attitude of the West towards Central Europe — towards the East, that is, to establish economic relations with the East, to look for markets in the East for the produce of Central Europe. Since we have become used to seeing everything in economic terms, the pattern is extended eastwards.

But such a view is in fact completely out of touch with reality. And that is why I spoke earlier about the way that the East and the West are involved in the whole of modern civilization, in order to create a basis for making a judgement about these things. The question is, simply: are the influential business people who are part of that configuration which, influenced by economic considerations, accepts what continues to be called the 'German Reich' correct when they say that economic relations as such should be directly established with the East?

Those who think about the question in abstract terms, as is common today, will say: yes! But anyone who takes account of what the cultural, political and economic life of the nineteenth century and the most recent age in general has taught us will probably reach a different conclusion. For let us just take the facts as they really exist. We have plenty of opportunity to see with what devotion and how gladly the Eastern part of Europe accepts the Central European cultural life if we look at the relationship as it developed in the nineteenth century into its last decades. For if you look at the cultural life of Russia and ask yourself how it arose you will see that two things are alive in it.

First of all, in true Russian cultural life, in all the things which approach us from there and which have been taken in by Central Europe in the last decades of the nineteenth century with a certain sensationalism, we do indeed encounter the reflexes of good Central European thinking. With great willingness, more than in Germany itself, the German thinkers and everything connected with German thinking was accepted in Russia. In the first half of the nineteenth century, in particular, Germans were recruited to set up Russian education in very concrete terms. It is evident everywhere how those things which exist as concrete ideas and intentions with regard to Russian institutions arose as the result of influences from Central Europe, and specifically German personalities, influences which arose in the same way as the legendary Rurik rulers. In relation to them one keeps hearing it said that the Russians had all kinds of different things but no order. That is why they turned to the three brothers and asked them to create order. That is roughly what it was like throughout the whole of the nineteenth century in relation to all those things which exist as the sources of culture in the relationship to Central Europe. In all situations where something was needed to assimilate specific things, in all those situations Russia turned to Central Europe or Western Europe. But the reaction to the two areas was quite different. Central European life was assimilated into Russian life with a certain ease, without much fuss, and continued to exist. The cultural life which came more from Western Europe was assimilated with a great deal of fuss so that it took on specific, sensational features, that it was integrated with certain pomp and decorative element. That is something which must be taken into account. Take the important Russian philosopher Solovyev. Such a philosopher had quite a different meaning in a Russian context as a philosopher coming from a Central European context. All his thinking is Central European, Hegelian, Kantian or Goetheanistic, and so on. We find a reflection of our own life everywhere when we study the specific thoughts of this philosopher. We can even go as far as to say that the specific thoughts in Tolstoy are Central European or Western European — but with all the differences that I have just explained. The same applies to Dostoyevsky, despite his stubborn adherence to Russian national chauvinism. All of that is the one aspect.

But you can notice a certain unified rejection in Russia when at the end of the nineteenth century and start of the twentieth century Russia was affected by the economic machinations of Central Europe. Just consider the way in which certain provisions in the trade treaties and suchlike were received. And consider the over-sensitive way in which the Russian element acted, apart from the noisy ones, the over-sensitive behaviour of Russia as a nation in the rejection of those things which manifested themselves as economic invasion or as economic expansion of power.

All of that should be understood as a signal. All of these things should show that it would be acting inappropriately if the objective today were to establish a relationship with the East through trade or other economic relations. The important thing which we must achieve despite the great difficulties associated with it through the Bolshevik element is to take to Russia the cultural element to the extent that it is based in productive culture. Everything generated by a productive culture affects views and emotions which concern the cultural life itself, or the life of the state or the economy. All of that is accepted quite well by the Russian element.

For the second element in addition to the first one, which really only consists of assimilating concrete German thinking in particular, the second element in Russian cultural life is a—how shall we call it?—an undifferentiated, vague (this is not meant in any provocative sense but is simply used as a term) a vague brew of emotions and feelings. It is this, for example, which can be observed quite characteristically in a philosopher who is quite typical of the Russian element such as Solovyev. His thoughts could not be more German, but they appear in quite a different form in Solovyev than they do in German thinkers. The Goethean element, too, appears in quite a different form in Solovyev. A certain brew of emotions and feelings is poured over it which gives the whole thing a certain nuance. But this nuance is the only thing which distinguishes this life. And this nuance is something passive, something accepting. And it is dependent on assimilating the Central European cultural life.

On the basis of this intercourse between the Central European cultural life and the Russian national element something magnificent can develop for the future. But one must have a feeling for the way in which such intercourse can build civilizations. However, it must occur in the purely cultural sphere. It must occur in a sphere which builds on the relationship between one person and another. It is this relationship which we must develop with the East. And once this is recognized, something will enter those things which develop on the basis of the cultural life which we might call a natural economic community. It must not be the starting-point because if it is it will be rejected. Everything which economists can achieve with regard to the East will lead to nothing if it is not built on the basis of what I have just explained. It is a key social question that this should be taken into consideration.

The other thing must be our relationship with the West. You see, it is impossible to instruct the West with those things which are our Central European cultural life. And this impossibility should clearly be taken into account — apart from the fact that it is already exceedingly difficult simply to translate what we think here in Central Europe, what we feel in Central Europe and what the East feels as well. The whole way of looking at things concerned with cultural matters is thoroughly different between the Central European areas on the one hand and the West and America on the other. People were surprised that Wilson understood so little of Europe when he came to Paris. They would have been less surprised if they had looked at a fat book that Wilson wrote as early as the 1890s called *The State*. That book was actually written wholly under the influence of European scholarship. But look at what this European scholarship turned into! If one had looked at the antecedents, the models, however, there would have been no surprise that Wilson was unable to understand a thing about matters European. He was not capable of that. For to the extent that we are talking about the thinking as such, to that extent it is a vain effort to try and produce a direct impression. In contrast, it would be quite significant to imagine the matter in the following terms, namely, to say that if one tries to negotiate with the West, nation to nation, there is not much joy to be had. But if the statesmen and scholars are excluded from the negotiations — scholars in all fields and statesman most of all — if not statesmen are sent to the West but only economists, then the people of the West will understand those economists with positive results. Only in the field of the economic life will there be any direct understanding in the West.

That does not mean, however, that one should restrict oneself only to the economic life in any intercourse with the West. No indeed, that is not necessary. It is, for example, most interesting to observe concert halls, large concert halls, in the western countries and to look at the names of famous composers displayed there: Mozart, Beethoven, Wagner and so on. As a rule, you will see only German names. So you can rest assured that if one wants to make an impression in the West solely on the basis of the substance of Central European thought, one would not get very far either with the Latin or the Anglo-Saxon element. That does not, of course, exclude talking with people there about what is being thought in Central Europe. Of course you can do that. But one must talk in a different way from Central Europe, where the life of ideas, of thoughts is the primary focus. Let us take a larger example. To a greater extent than what is generally today communicated as the ideas underlying our building in Dornach, Western Europeans and Americans have perhaps understood the building itself, those things which have resulted as concrete facts from the whole undertaking.

Of course one can give the matter itself a form in presenting it which allows the factual elements to emerge. Thus we got to a stage before the war—we can highlight this without being immodest—that I was able to give a German lecture in Paris in May 1914 which had to be translated word for word but I was able to give it in German. And this lecture, I state this as a fact only, was more successful than any lecture I ever gave in Germany. We had reached a stage where that was possible. But in such a case it is necessary to transform what is being said in a very specific way so that it is presented to people to a greater extent with the façade, with the artistic element, with those things which it becomes, which have an external effect. Here the 'how' is very important.

And that is why it is not at all unrealistic but a very concrete and real thought to say that we will make a big impression in the West if we understand our task properly in this way, if we really move beyond those things in which we cannot and will never succeed because we will never do them as well as the West, if we move beyond an imitation of the West. It does not matter whether we copy machines from the West—we will never build them as exactly as the West—or whether we imitate false teeth from the West, we will never make them as elegant. It does not really matter what it is! If we simply imitate we will never cope with the West because it does not need to take what we produce. But if we grasp what we can do and what the West cannot, if, for example, we were to imbue technology with art and artistic understanding, if we really achieved what has long figured in our Anthroposophical Society but what we cannot implement because we do not have the right people who are willing to do it, if, for example, we were to design locomotives artistically, if we were to design the stations artistically, if we were to give our characteristics to those things which we can take hold of, then western people would accept it and they would understand it. And then they would also interact with us. But we have to have some idea of what such interaction should be. Each person has to do that in their own field but it must be done. And a start has to be made in the present by recognizing how the threefolding impulse arises from the concrete conditions.

We must have a cultural life which is constituted such that it can have an effect in the East as I have just described; only a productive cultural life can do that. With it we could easily outdo all those Lunacharskys and the others. Because in the long term they would not be able to enslave the Russian people, the Russian folk soul. Once we have such a productive cultural life, it will happen that we will make an impression on the East. We must simply become strong enough to make such a cultural life count. We must overcome all these terrible people who are trying to stamp on cultural life in order to kill it.

We have, after all, reached such a stage in the hostility against the cultural life that I recently had to read out a passage in Dornach in which the author said that enough spiritual sparks had been ignited in the conflict with spiritual science and that the time was overdue for real sparks to ignite the Dornach building. Our opponents are assuming the most brutal forms. The key thing is to make the productive cultural life count and to ignore people's taunts and whatever else they do. Because it is possible to know that this productive cultural life, which can arise in Central Europe, can call forth a great fraternity which can extend to the East and can unite the East with Central Europe, whereas all brutal economic machinations would only create more and more rifts between Central Europe and the East. It is exceedingly important that such things should be understood and popularized. After all, it is important for the reason alone that if a wide public is won over for such things people begin to think differently about the remaining social questions as well, once they have started to think along those lines.

But it must happen on a broader basis than has been the case hitherto. It is necessary to work with real energy to ensure that the things we do are not, in a certain sense, lost causes. For it must be stressed, my dear friends, that there is plenty of material available in our threefolding newspaper but it is still imprisoned in a certain sense because it is only the written word so far. This requires constant work. But that is not always possible. In reality, the things that are initiated in various places must be worked on by many people on a broad basis. A clear view of these things is required.

We must be quite clear that we need a free, productive cultural life and that we have to cultivate it so that we can enter a possible relationship with the East.

And equally, we must have an economic life in which the state does not interfere, in which the cultural life does not interfere, in which only business people negotiate with the West in the first instance. Such negotiations must be conducted only by business people. That is the only way to achieve a positive result. One can and should negotiate with the West at state level for as long as no other possibility exists. But nothing much of use will come of it. Something useful will only begin to emerge when our politicians disappear from the economic negotiations irrespective of the response from those on the other side. Let politicians from the other side negotiate! There politicians are involved in the economic life. But when business people over here become politicians they lose their economic capacities, they think only in terms of the state.

The key thing is to understand the real demands of life. For that reason alone we need a threefold division of the social organism so that we can send business people to the West who are not influenced by the machinations of the state and cultural life. And we need a free cultural life so that we can establish a feasible relationship with the East. The international situation itself creates such a need.

How that is organized in detail must be left to each person to work out for himself. Because I only want to indicate here the direction in which we need to move. But it is an indication based on the reality of the situation. And the things which have been repeatedly stated should be taken with profound seriousness. It is not true that the practitioners really understand something of practical life. Basically they do not understand a thing about practical life — particularly if they are practitioners. This is because today's practitioners are really dependent on theory to the largest extent because they completely immerse themselves in theoretical thought structures in their practice. That is precisely what must be properly understood in the most profound sense of the word. And we must boldly base our so-called 'agitation' on circumstances as they really exist.

We must, above all, be clear that modern economic life

as such produces the need for threefolding. And it does so because this economic life is today a chaotic mixture of impulses from the East, impulses from the West and impulses from the middle. Basically the economic life consists of three elements: of the products of nature as we have discussed in the previous hour; then of those things produced by people's work; and finally of the product of capital. Capital, human work and the products of nature which are then processed further in production are what figure in the economic life.

And just as the threefold human organism consists of three components, which are in turn subject to a threefold division, the same applies to the social organism.[54] The head is certainly a human organ which is primarily a nervous and sensory organ; but the head also receives nourishment, it is, in a certain sense, penetrated by organs of nourishment. Equally, we have something of the nervous and sensory organism in the metabolic organism and serving it. This is the sympathetic nervous system. The same applies to the threefold division of the social organism. Each of the three components in turn contain the whole. But today it exists in an inorganic fashion, in a way which destroys life rather than builds it up.

First of all, we have nature, and production is, after all, only an extension of nature. And to the extent that nature is involved, our economic life still contains a very eastern experience, wholly from the East. It will not occur to eastern people that human labour is something that should belong to the economic life. And even if we go back to our earlier economic circumstances, which were still governed by eastern conditions, you will never find that human labour figures in the economic life.

And it is, indeed, something impossible that human labour should figure in the economic life.[55] For you can add apples and apples and you will get a total of some kind. And you can also add apples and pears as fruit and get a result. But I cannot see how you can add apples and glasses for example and get a common total. Now the content of goods, of a product, is fundamentally different from what has flowed into the product as human labour, as the Marxists say, which is a foolish way to describe it, although it is a popular one today. To make human labour and what constitutes goods, products, into something that is the same is as great a nonsense as wanting to make apples and spectacles into something common. But modern economics has done precisely that. The economic life has thus managed the feat of eating the spectacles, as it were, and taking the apples as an aid for better vision.

People do not notice these things in human life. It is noticed in subordinate realms of nature. It sounds paradoxical to say it, but that is what happens constantly. And by having wages in economic life at all, and wages must be paid and contain something which is included in the price of the goods in the same way that the goods contain products of nature, we have indeed added apples and spectacles. It is an impossibility. It is inconceivable.

When these three areas of the social organism — culture, the state and the law, and the economy — were still regulated on the basis of ancient conditions (the latter in an eastern way), when production was based on using surpluses without much thought being devoted to it (I compared it in the previous session to being little higher than the animals which also take no more than what nature offers), goods and labour were not combined in our regions either in ancient times. Work was regulated in a different way. One might be a lord whose social position was inherited from his forebears. If such blood did not flow in one's veins, one might be bonded labour, a serf or a slave. In other words, people's relationships were governed by laws. Whether one had to work or whether one could take it easy and watch others working was not determined by price or monetary relationships but was based on juridical relationships. Work was regulated on quite a different basis than the traffic in goods. That was kept quite separate in such organization based on ancient circumstances, something which is no longer of use to us today. There were two things in the East: goods and human labour. It was always considered that the juridical labour conditions were determined on a different basis from the circulation of goods. True, the former were based on these old juridical conditions. But labour was not paid in some way but rather a person would be assigned a position and would work, and the product of his work circulated. But human labour did not 'suffuse' the product in some way.

As you can see, the things created in the economy by labour already contain a juridical, state relationship through such labour. When we refer to the purely economic elements in the economy we are referring to goods and commodities. But as soon as we refer to the developed economy, that is, the economy based on the division of labour, we have to take a state and juridical element into account so that labour regulation belongs to the state and juridical sphere. It thus impacts on the other element of the social organism. And capital—capital essentially belongs to that relationship in the economic life which supports the economy culturally. Capital is what creates the economic centres, the enterprises. It is the cultural element in the economic life. But under modern materialism such cultural life in the economy has assumed a materialistic character. However, it is nevertheless the cultural life in the economy. The capitalist element is the spirit in the economic life.

This leads us, in turn, to look for a threefold structure in the economy itself. In other words, what flows into the actual economy—in which goods are produced, circulate and consumed—as labour must be associated with the sphere of rights and the state; and capital, which is actually the cultural element, must be associated with the cultural life. You can find this set out in concrete terms in *Towards Social Renewal* where it says that the transfer of capital, the circulation of capital must have a specific relationship to the cultural life. This is the key thing that we learn to keep these three areas separate in the economy.

But we will only have a true picture of the actual

situation if we are aware on the one hand that we have in a
certain respect to regulate what people from the East
simply ignored — the relationship between human economic life and nature. Among the people of the East it was
self-evident. We have to regulate it. In western people, the
whole of the cultural life, as I explained it earlier, was
subsumed in the economy. Even Spencer thinks in economic terms when he allegedly thinks scientifically. It is
all caught up in the economic life. Culture has acquired
features of the economy. That is why capitalism as such
turns materialistic. Capital is needed, as it says in *Towards
Social Renewal*, but the way that the spirit in the cultural
sphere is concentrated in capital will encounter the
greatest resistance in the West where capitalism, as it is
currently constituted, corresponds precisely to the western way of thinking in which everything of a spiritual
nature descends into the material. That is why basically
everything which is now imposed on the centre by the
West, on which many unjustified words have been spent,
is basically nothing more than the effect of western
capitalism writ large. So that people believe they are
dealing with a state structure whereas the Western states
have in fact become subject to capitalist influences. So they
are not pure state structures. The statesmen there are
basically economists just as the academics are. And so
these things will have to be kept apart — things which, on
the one hand, we have to penetrate with thought in economic life and which the East is not used to penetrating
with thinking, and which on the other hand have to be

penetrated with spirit with regard to capitalism while the West shows not the slightest inclination to penetrate these things with spirit. These things are the task of the Central European regions. That is also why something was created in these Central European areas which we will now scrutinize very closely.

It happens repeatedly—here in Stuttgart and in Switzerland, and friends elsewhere have experienced similar things—that people say: even if we agree with the division into a free cultural life and a free economic life, nothing remains for the state! Indeed, in the form which the state is constituted today, the way it has absorbed the cultural life which does not belong there, on the one hand, and sucks up more and more of the economic life, on the other, the actual life of the state itself withers away. The actual life of the state, those things which take place from person to person, between all adult persons, no longer exists. That is why the only thing that people, such as the law professor Rudolf Stammler and his followers, can say is that the state exists to give the economy its form. But it is precisely the point that the state will only arise in the appropriate way and encompass all those things which take place between people purely by the fact that they are people—and this includes the whole field of labour relations—when the other sectors are separated off. Only when that has happened will a truly democratic state be able to develop. It is hardly surprising that today there is still no proper concept of this kind of state because there is still no proper concept of an independent democracy because people only think in abstract terms and rush into a definition of democracy. Definition, of course, is no problem. Definition always reminds me of the ancient Greek example, which I have often quoted, where someone quite properly defines the human being as a living being which walks on two legs and does not have feathers. The next day the speaker was presented with a plucked goose and was told: so this is a human being because it walks on two legs and has no feathers. Definitions can be used for all kinds of purposes. But we are not dealing with definitions, we need to find the realities.

Take the concept of democracy as it exists today, which is basically of western origin. How did it arise? You can study the development of England and its more ancient reigns and you will find that there is an endeavour to shake off bondage. But it has a religious character which becomes particularly pronounced under Cromwell. Something develops on the basis of the theocratic and puritan element, of the freedom of religion, which is then separated out from theocracy, from belief, and which turns into the democratic and political element of freedom. That is what is described as a sense of democracy in the West. It is separated from the independent sense of religion. Here we have a real concept of democracy. And there will not be a real concept of democracy until a separate organization exists between the cultural and economic organization which is based solely on the relationship between people and the equality of all people. Only then will a state relationship result.

It is a characteristic feature that ideas have arisen in Central Europe, without this leading to threefolding, which pose the question: how should the state be created? It is highly interesting that Wilhelm von Humboldt, who became a Prussian minister (a peculiar affair in itself), wrote a beautiful essay in the first half of the nineteenth century called *The Limits of State Action*[56] which is based on certain ideas from Schiller and Goethe. He genuinely endeavours to discover how it might be possible to build the state, to define in the social conditions what belongs purely to the state, politics, law. Wilhelm von Humboldt did not completely succeed in doing so but that is not the important thing. His ideas should have been developed. And while we fail to create what is real with regard to the state, while Stammler and his ilk say that the life of the state only exists to provide a form for the economic life, we will not get any further. These things need to be presented extensively to a wider public today and it needs to happen fast. For only by introducing healthy thinking to our contemporaries and spreading these thoughts as quickly as possible can we make any progress.

The opposing forces are strong. They jeer and apply their destructive forces from all quarters. And there should be no illusion about the strong purpose which exists on that side. For if the move which we are now undertaking is to have any meaning, it has to be on the understanding that we have tried to establish a social impulse on the basis of anthroposophically oriented spiritual science. After all, anthroposophically oriented spiritual science can take its time, can progress slowly, can take account of what people can cope with. Cliques may form here too. But these cliques exist only in the physical world; the spiritual movement leaves them behind. The true life force which underlies the real anthroposophical movement has its meaning, its content in the spiritual world. It is not really that important whether cliques form or whether there are sectarian traits and so on. These are of course things which have to be fought individually one by one in our so serious time. But these things are not as bad as the wrong action being undertaken in the field where the practical element, those things which will have an immediate effect, has to be derived from the anthroposophical movement, those things as they exist in what we might call the social wing of the anthroposophical movement. Here there is no time to wait. Here we cannot set up associations for threefolding that are organized in such a way that they merely reflect the old anthroposophical branches. Here we have to be clear that what we fail to develop until tomorrow, be it ever so good, may well be worse than what we develop today even if it is not quite as good. Here it is essential to act strongly directly in the present, here and now, and that to wait a day may produce a result which comes a day too late. And we can, indeed, see from events how things are happening too late from week to week. That is why the action which we are about to undertake was initiated and that is why we think it is so important, because it is necessary for things to happen quickly. Europe cannot afford to lose any more time.

What is needed now is to make people think in a way

that allows reality to play a role in such thinking. Humanity has basically been educated in such a way that a completely unrealistic way of thinking is what matters in practical life. It is an unrealistic way of thinking when people stand up today and say that rights need to be cultivated, that we should progress in some way in social life from an ethical standpoint. These things are very nice of course, but they are very abstract. Spiritual aspects are only of value if they interact directly with physical life, if they can really support and overcome material aspects. Otherwise they are of no value whatsoever. We should not be taken in by the harangues of Förster or people like him. They sound very nice but they do not penetrate material life because the people who harangue us have no understanding of material life but believe that preaching will somehow advance today's material world.

And that is the mistake made by the bourgeoisie. It has steadily withdrawn into its own realm of luxury as far as the life of the soul is concerned. For six days a week it sits in its office. The accounts ledger may have 'God be with us!' written at the front, but there is very little of God on the following pages. 'God be with us!' is very abstract. And then, having worked all week in the way that we know so well, it goes to church to listen to a sermon full of spiritual lust about eternal salvation. In other words, it turns spiritual life into a luxury and deprives material life of the spirit. The bourgeoisie has achieved great advances in this respect. It has pushed further and further so that in the end all of spiritual life has indeed become an ideology.

It is hardly surprising, then, if the proletariat comes along and in turn declares on a theoretical basis that the spirit is ideology and then attempts to restructure the whole of the economy purely from the perspective of the means of production. Both things belong together. Things have truly reached a stage today in which the battle between the bourgeoisie and the proletariat consists only of the extent to which the one is at the bottom and the other on top and vice versa. It is no more than a battle. There is no intention to achieve a productive development of life by penetrating the issues more deeply. That can only be done if one has a more comprehensive impulse that comprises the human being as a whole.

But in such an event one either has to concern oneself with threefolding, if one agrees with it, or one must be capable of replacing threefolding with something better. All the other things manifesting themselves today fail to take the human being as such into account in any way at all. That is why our movement needs to be rescued, we might say, soonest from the intentions of our opponents. Their purpose is to make our movement impossible through their machinations. And these machinations have now become very sophisticated. Just think of the sophistication in the campaign now being waged by the *Berliner Tageblatt* newspaper. The *Berliner Tageblatt* fabricates an article which mentions all kinds of daft 'occultists' and in the middle of it refers to anthroposophy which has nothing whatsoever to do with them. But this saves people from having to grasp what anthroposophy is about because they can simply file it away under this rubbish. Of course the rubbish written there is not difficult to understand and people have no further need to look at anthroposophy in particular. These things happen internationally too, we can see it everywhere, in English newspapers, everywhere. But that is only the one thing. In the near future a campaign is starting—has already started, but is being continued—to destroy what our movement stands for. That is why we must recall today what needs to be done. And if something decisive fails to happen on a broad basis then we have no option but to acknowledge that we have an idea of what could be done on the basis of anthroposophically oriented spiritual science also in respect of society but we do not have the strength to put it into practice. If we see the strength of purpose with which the opposing side works, sometimes a strength of purpose fuelled by wicked intent, we have to understand that we must generate a similar purpose. They want to achieve a bad purpose so why can we not generate the same strength for a good one? Why should anyone be able to say with justification that here we had the intention to produce something of benefit to humankind; but the opposition was something quite different, it had strength of purpose and it was willing to put that purpose into action.

My dear friends, if we do not occupy the ground on which we can put our purpose into action, we will of course fail to achieve anything at the present time. In a certain respect, we are currently in an either/or situation

in our movement. That is why this action was introduced.
I would ask you to reflect on that. I would ask you to make
that part of your purpose before we move on to develop
what we need for that purpose.

Notes

1   W.F. Lofthouse, *London Quarterly Review*, January 1923.

2   *New York Times Review of Books*, 14 January 1923; *Journal of Political Economy*, 1923; *American Economic Review*, January 1924.

3   In Rudolf Steiner, *Reincarnation and Immortality*, Multimedia Publishing Corp., 1970, pp. 173–204.

4   Rudolf Steiner Press, 1972.

5   Anthroposophic Press, 1985.

6   Rudolf Steiner Press, 1992.

7   *World Economy*, lecture of 29 July 1922, Rudolf Steiner Press.

8   This has not been translated. The German source is *Uber die Dreigliederung des sozialen Organismus*, GA 24, Rudolf Steiner Verlag, Dornach, Switzerland, 1982.

9   Part of this passage is taken from *The Life and Work of Rudolf Steiner*, by Guenther Wachsmuth, Whittier Books, New York, 1955, p. 316. The remainder is from a copy of the original German MS.

10   Wilson did not introduce his 14-point proposal until January 1918. Two other dates worth mentioning are 6 April 1917, when the US entered the war against Germany after Germany sank a ship without regard to flag, and 11 March 1917, when the Russian Revolution began.

11   Two contemporary works that also provide useful background are *In the Name of the New World Order* by Amnon Reuveni and *Mapping the Millennium* by Terry Boardman, both published by Temple Lodge Publishing. Steiner's two-

volume cycle of lectures *The Karma of Untruthfulness* is also essential reading (Rudolf Steiner Press).

12   In *Light for the New Millennium*, edited by Thomas Meyer, Rudolf Steiner Press, 1997.

13   For the story of Steiner's failed attempt to introduce von Moltke's memoir at the Treaty of Versailles see *Light for the New Millennium*, edited by Thomas Meyer, Rudolf Steiner Press, 1997. Steiner had hoped that the participants at the treaty conference would not have ratified the treaty with the war guilt clause had they learned the information in the von Moltke memoir.

14   In *From Symptom to Reality in Modern History* (Rudolf Steiner Press, 1976) Steiner presents his approach to studying history. In this approach the historian looks for events that are symptoms of the deeper driving forces of historical developments. History can be illuminated by depicting a sequence of leading symptoms that illuminate the historic landscape as mighty lightning flashes that make visible what otherwise is dark.

15   In his memoir, von Moltke revealed the shocking fact that because the Kaiser was so loose-lipped he was not even informed of the details of the Schlieffen Plan.

16   I am told by the British historian Terry Boardman that 'public opinion' at that time referred to the views of an elite circle of media editors, club members and parliamentarians, and not as it does today to the views of the general public as indicated by statistical opinion polls.

17   *British Documents on the Origins of the War, 1898–1914*, Vol. XI, edited by G.P. Gooch and Harold Temperley, 1926.

18   Lindisfarne Press, 1993.

19   The year Bismark consolidated the modern German state.

20 *Light for the New Millennium,* edited by Thomas Meyer, Rudolf Steiner Press, London, 1997, pp. 93–100.

21 See Stephen E. Usher's introduction to *The Esoteric Aspect of the Social Question; The Individual and Society* by Rudolf Steiner (Rudolf Steiner Press, London, 2001) for details of Hitler's written attack and the attempt on Steiner's life.

22 Arthur Polzer-Hoditz wrote an excellent book about the short reign of the young Emperor, *The Emperor Karl,* Putnam, London, 1930. The German edition of 1929 includes a full account of the memorandum that reached the Emperor and the memorandum is included in the appendix of the volume. The English edition neatly removes all reference to Steiner, the threefold social order and the memorandum.

23 Hans Kuehn, *Dreigliederungs-Zeit,* Philosophisch-Anthroposophischer Verlag, Goetheanum, Dornach, Switzerland, 1978, p. 18.

24 In *Towards Social Renewal,* Chapter 4, p. 139. Also see *The Challenge of the Times,* Rudolf Steiner, Anthroposophic Press, New York, 1941, lecture of 29 November 1918.

25 There are deeper, esoteric aspects to the fact that von Baden stood in this remarkable position in world history. That Max von Baden was the head of the house of Baden was a consequence of the crime against Kaspar Hauser in the early part of the nineteenth century. Hauser was born the heir of the house of Baden in 1812 and, according to a remark related to Steiner, was destined to become a significant figure in Central European history. Poltzer-Hoditz described it thus: 'Southern Germany should have become the new Grail Castle of the new Knights of the Grail and the cradle of future events. The spiritual ground had been well prepared by all those personalities we know of as Goethe,

Schiller, Hölderlin, Herder and others. Kaspar Hauser was to have gathered around him, as it were, all that existed in this spiritual ground thus prepared.' (See *Kaspar Hauser* by Peter Tradowsky, Temple Lodge, 1997.) Hauser's activity would have prepared the ground for the threefold social order. But Hauser's destiny was crossed by the activity of occultists intent on stopping him. He was abducted from the cradle. Knowing that if he were immediately killed he would quickly reincarnate, the abductors imprisoned the infant in dark cellars where he was kept, without any human contact, until he was about 15 years old. He was then released into a town square in Nuremberg, his captors expecting him to vanish from the historic scene as a kind of retarded individual. But he was found by people who grasped the nature of the crime that had been committed. With much care and tutoring he gained the ability to speak and then to write. When it became apparent that he might be recognized for who he was he was murdered in 1833 at the age of 21. The house of Baden passed into the hands of other people as a consequence of the crime and Max von Baden eventually became the heir of the house. That von Baden found himself in the world historic situation where he might have brought the threefold social order into existence in middle Europe at this critical juncture in history was thus an event of world historic significance.

26   It is my understanding that Steiner had hoped that von Baden would have emerged as a leading figure in a new German government with the will to lead a transformation of old state structure in the direction of the threefold idea and that the emperor Karl would have played a similar role in Austro-Hungary.

27   Lecture of 21 and 22 February 1920 from *Ideas for a New Europe*, Rudolf Steiner Press, 1992.

28   In *Towards Social Renewal*, Rudolf Steiner Press.

29   *A Theory of Knowledge Based on Goethe's World Conception*, Anthroposophic Press, 1968. The original German volume is *Grundlinien einer Erkenntnistheorie der Goetheschen Weltanschauung*, GA 2. It was originally published in 1886.

30   This translation was published first in *The Threefold Review*, Summer/Autumn, Issue No. 9. The original German texts are found in *Methodische Grundlagen der Anthroposophie, Gesammelte Aufsatze zur Philosophie, Naturwissenschaft, Aesthetik und Seelenkunde 1884–1901*, GA 30, Rudolf Steiner Verlag, Dornach, Switzerland, 1989.

31   Henry Thomas Buckle, 1821–62.

32   The English text was first published in *The Threefold Review*, Winter/Spring 1994/94 (Issue No. 10). The German text is found in *Beiträge zur Rudolf Steiner Gesamtausgabe*, 1985, No. 88. The text is the manuscript of a lecture delivered by Steiner on 26 October 1905.

33   Crimmitschau strikes: among the numerous work stoppages in the first years of the twentieth century, the strike of the textile workers of Crimmitschau from 7 August 1903 to 17 January 1904 stands out especially because the management reacted to the strike of 600 textile workers in five factories with an unprecedented mass lockout — they locked out the entire work force. Subsequently, in Crimmitschau, with a population of 23,000, around 8000 textile workers and 1500 who worked at home stood in conflict with a management that was obviously intensifying its measures against the workers. For details on this strike see F. Deppe et al., *Geschichte der deutschen Gewerkschaftsbewegung* (History of

the German Trade Union Movement), Cologne, 1978, p. 77f. Miners' strike: a further high point in the strike movement was the miners' strike in the Ruhr from December 1904 to 9 February 1905, at the centre of which stood the demands for an eight-hour day, higher pay, better worker protection, and recognition of the workers' organizations. For this also see the portrayal of F. Deppe et al., op cit., p. 78f.

What is going on in Eastern Europe: on 22 August 1905, 'Bloody Sunday'. In Petersburg, peaceful demonstrators were shot down by the military. The strike wave now turned into revolutionary unrest that soon spread over all of Russia. In the autumn of 1905 the socialistically organized workers called for a general strike and with the participation of Bolsheviks, Mensheviks, social revolutionaries and independents formed the first Soviet (Council).

34   Alfred Kolb: Rudolf Steiner also deals with him in the essay 'Spiritual Science and the Social Question' in *Lucifer Gnosis*, GA 134, and in the Hamburg lecture of the same name of 2 March 1908 in *Die Welträtsel und die Anthroposophie* (Riddles of the World and Anthroposophy), GA 54.

35   Square brackets indicate insertions by the German editor.

36   The world-view of Ernst Haeckel (1834–1919), German naturalist and philosopher.

37   For a characterization of intuition as used by Steiner, see, for example, his essays from 1905, *The Stages of Higher Knowledge*.

38   The German *drei Stadien* translates to 'three stages'. We suggest this represents a stenographic error and take the liberty of correcting it for the sake of clarity.

39   Social democracy is 'a political theory advocating the use of democratic means to achieve a gradual transition from

capitalism to socialism'. *American Heritage Dictionary*, 1992. Social Democrat (with capitals) refers to a member of the Social Democratic Party (SDP) in Germany, which was founded in the late nineteenth century.

40   Refers to the first fundamental principle of the Theosophical Society: 'To form a nucleus of the universal brotherhood of humanity without distinction of race, creed, sex, caste or colour.'

41   Claude Henri de Rouvroy Saint-Simon, 1760–1825: social reformer. *Lettres d'un habitant de Genève à ses contemporains* (Letters of an Inhabitant of Geneva to his Contemporaries) (1803); *Réorganisations de la société européenne* (The Reorganization of European Society) (1814); *Le nouveau christianisme* (The New Christianity) (1825). Also see A. Voigt, *Die sozialen Utopien* (Social Utopias), Leipzig, 1906. This book is also to be found in Rudolf Steiner's private library (Archives of the Rudolf Steiner Estate Administration) and contains numerous underlinings by him concerning Saint-Simon. See p. 107ff.

42   François Marie Charles Fourier, 1772–1837. *Théorie des quatre mouvements et des destinées générales* (Theory of Four Movements and General Destinies) (1808); *Le nouveau monde industriel et sociétair* (The New Industrial and Societal World) (1829). See A. Voigt op. cit. p. 95ff.

43   Literally it says: 'I was also completely convinced that any great revolution is never the fault of the people, rather of the government. Revolutions are altogether impossible as long as governments are continually just and continually vigilant, so that they anticipate them with timely reforms and do not hold back until what is necessary is compelled from the bottom up' (Eckermann, 4 January 1824).

44   The original German texts are published in *Über die Drei-gliederung des sozialen Organismus und zur Zeitlage Shriften und Aufsätze 1915–1921*, Rudolf Steiner Verlag, 1982.

45   Letter of 22 May 1917 from Woodrow Wilson to the provisional government of Russia.

46   Ibid.

47   The German text is found in *Die soziale Grundforderung unserer Zeit*, GA 186, Rudolf Steiner Verlag, Dornach, Switzerland, 1990.

48   Steiner's world-view includes a view of ages of history and of the evolution of human consciousness through these ages. The most recent ages are what he calls the 'cultural epochs'. These are periods of about 2200 years and are designated: 1. Ancient India, 2. Ancient Persia, 3. Egyptian, 4. Graeco-Roman, 5. fifth post-Atlantean, 6. sixth post-Atlantean, and 7. seventh post-Atlantean. The cultural epochs begin after the great flood that ended the civilization of Atlantis. Individual human beings tend to incarnate twice during each cultural epoch, once as a man and once as a woman. During each epoch humanity develops a certain aspect of its potential. In the Egyptian period humanity developed what Steiner refers to as the sentient soul, during the Graeco-Roman age the intellectual soul, during the fifth post-Atlantean period the spiritual soul (also translated as consciousness soul) and during the sixth post-Atlantian period the Spirit Self. The sentient soul is the part of the soul that is directed towards the world of the senses and the soul's likes and dislikes within that realm. The intellectual soul is a more inward aspect of the human being where he elaborates his experiences of the sense world, unlike the sentient soul that

tends to live more in the moment savouring its experiences. The intellectual soul allows the human being to enter into ideas of the good, the true and the beautiful. Steiner describes the difference between the consciousness soul and the Spirit Self as follows in his work *Theosophy* (Anthroposophic Press, 1971): 'The difference between the Spirit Self and the consciousness soul can be made clear in the following way. The consciousness soul is in touch with the self-existent truth that is independent of all antipathy and sympathy. The Spirit Self bears within it the same truth, but taken up into and enclosed by the 'I', individualized by it, and absorbed into the independent being of the individual. It is through the eternal truth becoming thus individualized and bound up into one being with the 'I' that the 'I' itself attains to the eternal.'

49   The Guardian of the Threshold, in Steiner's world-view, is a spiritual being that has no physical body and which the human being meets when he attempts to expand his consciousness to include experiences of the spiritual world beyond the world of the senses and the intellectual life connected with it. In this encounter with the Guarian of the Threshold the human being is given deep self-knowledge that is typically very difficult to endure but which is essential to the human being if he is to conduct himself rightly in the spiritual world. See for example Steiner's *Occult Science, An Outline*, Chapter 5.

50   See *Mapping the Millennium* by Terry Boardman, Temple Lodge, 1998, for a discussion of the maps to which Steiner referred.

51   From 1902 to 1912 Rudolf Steiner was the General Secretary of the German section of the Theosophical Society. He broke

with the Theosophical Society in 1912 and founded the Anthroposophical Society.

52 Published in English in *The Threefold Review*, Summer/ Autumn 1996 (Issue No. 4). The original German text is published in *Über die Dreigliederung des sozialen Organismus*, Rudolf Steiner Verlag, 1982.

53 Original German text from, *Wie wirkt man für den Impuls der Dreigliederung des sozialen Organismus?*, GA 338, Rudolf Steiner Verlag, 1986.

54 In his book *Towards Social Renewal*, Steiner compares the threefold social organism to the human organism. The economic life, the political life, and the cultural life correspond respectively to the nervous and sensory system, the system of circulation and respiration, and the system of metabolism and limbs. Here Steiner is observing that just as there is a metabolic process in the head so also is there a cultural process in the economic life, etc.

55 Here Steiner is developing the argument that labour cannot be treated like a commodity in economic life. But this is exactly what is done in modern economics where the concept of a market for labour is developed in a way exactly analogous to the concept of markets for commodities. In our contemporary way of thinking, a wage is the price of labour just as a certain sum is the price of a bushel of apples. Steiner argues that this is actually an impossible way of thinking as it compares incommensurate quantities. In his threefold social order the treatment of labour is a rights issue. See his *World Economy* or *Renewal of the Social Organism* for a detailed discussion of this issue.

56 Published by Liberty Fund, Indianapolis, IN, 1993.

Sources

1. 'Psychological Cognition' is a chapter from *A Theory of Knowledge Based on Goethe's World Conception*, Anthroposophic Press, 1968. It was originally published in German in 1886. The original texts are currently available in *Grundlinien einer Erkenntnistheorie der Goetheschen Weltanschauung*, GA 2, Rudolf Steiner Verlag, Dornach, Switzerland, 1979.

2. 'The Social Question' was published in three instalments in 1898 in *Das Magazin für Literatur* (No. 28, July 16, No. 29, July 23, and No. 30, July 30). This translation was published first in *The Threefold Review*, Summer/Autumn, Issue No. 9. The original German texts are found in *Methodische Grundlagen der Anthroposophie, Gesammelte Aufsätze zur Philosophie, Naturwissenschaft, Ästhetik und Seelenkunde 1884–1901*, GA 30, Rudolf Steiner Verlag, Dornach, Switzerland, 1989.

3. 'The Social Question and Theosophy' was first published in English in *The Threefold Review*, Winter/Spring 1993/94 (Issue No. 10). The German text is found in *Beiträge zur Rudolf Steiner Gesamtausgabe*, No. 88, St John's Tide, 1988, Rudolf Steiner Verlag, Dornach, Switzerland. The text is the manuscript of a lecture delivered by Steiner on 26 October 1905.

4. 'The Memoranda of 1917' are presented here for the first time in English. The original German texts are published in *Über die Dreigliederung des sozialen Organismus und zur Zeitlage Schriften und Aufsätze 1915–1921*, GA 24, Rudolf Steiner Verlag, Dornach, Switzerland, 1982.

5. 'The Metamorphosis of Intelligence' is a lecture of 15 December 1919 published in English for the first time in this volume. The German text is found in *Die soziale Grundforderung unserer Zeit*, GA 186, Rudolf Steiner Verlag, Dornach, Switzerland, 1990.

6. 'Culture, Law and Economy' was published in the newspaper *Soziale Zunkunft* in September 1919. It was published in English in *The Threefold Review,* Summer/Autumn 1996 (Issue No. 4). The original German text is published in *Über die Dreigliederung des sozialen Organismus,* GA 24, Rudolf Steiner Verlag, Dornach, Switzerland, 1982.

7. 'Central Europe between East and West' is published here for the first time in English. It is the text of a lecture Steiner delivered on the evening of 13 February 1921. The original German text is found in *Wie wirkt man für den Impuls der Dreigliederung des sozialen Organismus?,* GA 338, Rudolf Steiner Verlag, Dornach, Switzerland,1986.

Further Reading

On the threefold social order and related themes found in Rudolf Steiner's works:

Rudolf Steiner, *The Challenge of the Times*, Anthroposophic Press, New York, 1941.

Rudolf Steiner, *The Esoteric Aspects of the Social Question. The Individual and Society*, Rudolf Steiner Press, London, 2001.

Rudolf Steiner, *Ideas for a New Europe*, Rudolf Steiner Press, London, 1992.

Amnon Reuveni, *In the Name of the New World Order. Manifestations of Decadent Powers in World Politics*, Temple Lodge, London, 1996.

Peter Tradowsky, *Kaspar Hauser. The Struggle for the Spirit*, Temple Lodge, London, 1997.

Rudolf Steiner, *The Karma of Untruthfulness*, Vol. 1 and Vol. 2, Rudolf Steiner Press, London, 1988 and 1992.

Light for the New Millennium, Rudolf Steiner's Association with Helmuth and Eliza von Moltke, edited by T.H. Meyer, Rudolf Steiner Press, London, 1997.

Terry Boardman, *Mapping the Millennium. Behind the Plans of the New World Order*, Temple Lodge, 1998.

Rudolf Steiner, *The Mission of the Folk-Souls*, Rudolf Steiner Press, London, 1970.

Rudolf Steiner, *The Renewal of the Social Organism*, Anthroposophic Press, New York, 1985.

Rudolf Steiner, *Towards Social Renewal*, Rudolf Steiner Press, London, 1992.

Rudolf Steiner, *World Economy*, Rudolf Steiner Press, London, 1977.

Background reading:

Carroll Quigley, *The Anglo-American Establishment. From Rhodes to Cliveden*, Books In Focus, 1981.

John Maynard Keynes, *Economic Consequences of the Peace*, Harcourt, Brace and Howe, 1920.

Arthur Count Polzer-Hoditz, *The Emperor Karl*, Putnam, London, 1930.

Zbigniew Brzezinski, *The Grand Chessboard. American Primacy and Its Geostrategic Imperatives*, Basic Books, 1997.

James Joll, *The Origins of the First World War*, Longman, London, 1992.

Frederic C. Howe, *Socialized Germany*, Charles Scribner's Sons, New York, 1915.

Sigmund Freud and William C. Bullitt, *Thomas Woodrow Wilson. A Psychological Study*, Houghton Mifflin Company, Boston, 1966.

C.G. Harrison, *The Transcendental Universe*, Lindisfarne Press, New York, 1993.

Note Regarding Rudolf Steiner's Lectures

The lectures and addresses contained in this volume have been translated from the German, which is based on stenographic and other recorded texts that were in most cases never seen or revised by the lecturer. Hence, due to human errors in hearing and transcription, they may contain mistakes and faulty passages. Every effort has been made to ensure that this is not the case. Some of the lectures were given to audiences more familiar with anthroposophy; these are the so-called 'private' or 'members' lectures. Other lectures, like the written works, were intended for the general public. The difference between these, as Rudolf Steiner indicates in his *Autobiography*, is twofold. On the one hand, the members' lectures take for granted a background in and commitment to anthroposophy; in the public lectures this was not the case. At the same time, the members' lectures address the concerns and dilemmas of the members, while the public work speaks directly out of Steiner's own understanding of universal needs. Nevertheless, as Rudolf Steiner stresses: 'Nothing was ever said that was not solely the result of my direct experience of the growing content of anthroposophy. There was never any question of concessions to the prejudices and preferences of the members. Whoever reads these privately printed lectures can take them to represent anthroposophy in the fullest sense. Thus it was possible without hesitation — when the complaints in this direction became too persistent — to depart from the custom of circulating this material "For members only". But it must be borne in mind that faulty passages do occur in these reports not revised by myself.' Earlier in the same chapter, he states: 'Had I been able to correct them [the private lectures], the restriction *for members only* would have been unnecessary from the beginning.'

The original German editions on which this text is based were published by Rudolf Steiner Verlag, Dornach, Switzerland in the collected edition (*Gesamtausgabe*, 'GA') of Rudolf Steiner's work. All publications are edited by the Rudolf Steiner Nachlassverwaltung (estate), which wholly owns both Rudolf Steiner Verlag and the Rudolf Steiner Archive. The organization relies solely on donations to continue its activity.

For further information please contact:

Rudolf Steiner Archiv
Postfach 135
CH-4143 Dornach

or:

www.rudolf-steiner.com

ALSO AVAILABLE IN THE SAME SERIES:

AGRICULTURE

Compiled with an introduction, commentary and notes by
Richard Thornton Smith

The evolving human being; Cosmos as the source of life; Plants
and the living earth; Farms and the realms of nature; Bringing
the chemical elements to life; Soil and the world of spirit;
Supporting and regulating life processes; Spirits of the elements;
Nutrition and vitality; Responsibility for the future

ISBN 1 85584 113 4

ARCHITECTURE

Compiled with an introduction, commentary and notes by
Andrew Beard

The origins and nature of architecture; The formative influence
of architectural forms; The history of architecture in the light of
mankind's spiritual evolution; A new architecture as a means of
uniting with spiritual forces; Art and architecture as
manifestations of spiritual realities; Metamorphosis in
architecture; Aspects of a new architecture; Rudolf Steiner on the
first Goetheanum building; The second Goetheanum building;
The architecture of a community in Dornach; The temple is the
human being; The restoration of the lost temple

ISBN 1 85584 123 1

ART

Compiled with an introduction, commentary and notes by Anne Stockton

The being of the arts; Goethe as the founder of a new science of aesthetics; Technology and art; At the turn of each new millennium; The task of modern art and architecture; The living walls; The glass windows; Colour on the walls; Form—moving the circle; The seven planetary capitals of the first Goetheanum; The model and the statue 'The Representative of Man'; Colour and faces; Physiognomies

ISBN 1 85584 138 X

EDUCATION

Compiled with an introduction, commentary and notes by Christopher Clouder

A social basis for education; The spirit of the Waldorf school; Educational methods based on anthroposophy; The child at play; Teaching from a foundation of spiritual insight and education in the light of spiritual science; The adolescent after the fourteenth year; Science, art, religion and morality; The spiritual grounds of education; The role of caring in education; The roots of education and the kingdom of childhood; Address at a parents' evening; Education in the wider social context

ISBN 1 85584 118 5